THE AROMATIC DOG

ESSENTIAL OILS, HYDROSOLS & HERBAL OILS FOR EVERYDAY DOG CARE: A PRACTICAL GUIDE

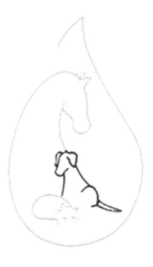

NAYANA MORAG

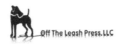

Off The Leash Press, LLC

Published by:
Off The Leash Press, LLC,
PO Box 275
Winter Park, FL 32790-0275
www.offtheleashpress.com
407-758-8309

First edition
Cover design © 2015 Rupa Bokhorst
Interior design by IndieDesignz.com
All interior photographs property of Nayana Morag.

Library of Congress Control number: 2015905795

LIBRARY OF CONGRESS CATALOGING-IN-PUBLICATION DATA
Morag, Nayana
The Aromatic Dog.Essential oils, hydrosols and herbal oils for everyday dog care:
A practical guide/by Nayana Morag
ISBN 978-0-9841982-6-9

1. Dogs-Health. 2. Dogs-Diseases-Alternative treatment.
3. Aromatherapy for Dogs. 4. Complementary Care. I. Title

Acknowledgements

Thanks go to:

Caroline Ingraham, with whom I trained and who pioneered the method of animal self-selection of essential oils.

Rupa Bokhorst for her useful insights as my "average dog owner" and her beautiful book cover.

Max Brecher for goading me to greater clarity.

Robin Moulsdale for his input and guidance.

Sherri Cappabianca from Off The Leash Press, for encouraging me to go into print again.

A big juicy bone goes to Thorling Thunderpaws our aromatic dog, who was a perfect model for the photos.

All the dogs who have contributed to my education and improved my listening skills. And as ever heart-felt thanks to my partner Prasado for everything he does to support me, body, and soul.

TABLE OF CONTENTS

INTRODUCTION

You love your dogs, and want them to live long, healthy, happy lives. You have heard that essential oils can be used to help you care for you dog more naturally, but where do you start?

I have developed a simple-to-follow system that is safe to use and gets great results.

With the help of this book you will discover how easy and economical it can be to use aromatics for your dog's well-being. I will share with you practical tips from my own experience of natural animal care and how I use aromatic extracts to:

- Solve simple health and behavior problems
- Calm nerves and increase trainability,
- Reduce stress, the major cause of disease, and
- Create a deeper bond between you and your much-loved dog.

I am a certified animal aromatherapist and have been teaching people how to use aromatic extracts for over 15 years. I love essential oils and don't know how anyone lives without them, especially if they have animals in their care.

Essential oils empower you. They allow you to care for your animals safely and easily. You can heal a wound without filling your dog full of antibiotics. You can prevent flea infestations without poisoning your dog with chemicals. You can keep your dog's immune system in tip-top condition so that the chances of infection are minimal.

But what I love most about essential oils, is that my dogs love them too. Allowing your dog to select his own medicine tells him you honor and respect him. This deepens your relationship. For me the art of listening is one of the secrets of good animal care. Watching your dog self-select aromatics teaches you to listen deeply.

Helping people and their dogs live healthy, harmonious lives together is my passion. This book is for all those of you who would like to use aromatic extracts (essential oils, hydrosols and vegetable oils) to keep your dogs brimming with vitality, from puppy-hood to old age.

Enjoy!

GETTING STARTED

Before we go any further, a quick look at the basic principles
and tools of the system

THE AROMATIC EXTRACTS

Essential oils

In nature, essential oils can be found in either the seeds, roots, leaves, resin, bark or flowers of aromatic plants. In different plants they have different functions; for example, to protect from microbes or attract insects for pollination.

They are most commonly extracted from the plant by steam distillation. Plant material is put in a large vat. Steam is then forced through under pressure, condensed and collected as water. The essential oil collects on top of the water and is separated out.

Essential oils are also produced using solvent extraction, in which case they are known as absolutes.

Essential oils are highly volatile, light weight and penetrative. They are easily absorbed through the skin or by breathing them in. Inhaling an essential oil brings it directly into the regions of the brain concerned with emotions and memory. The nervous system transforms the messages from the aromatic chemicals into physical responses in the body, such as the anti-inflammatory, relaxation or anti-allergenic responses.

Essential oils are mostly produced for the fragrance and flavoring industries, which demand high yield and low cost and produce inferior quality oil. Essential oils suitable for therapeutic use are distilled with care, slowly and at a lower temperature, so more of the healing molecules remain intact.

Unfortunately, many essential oils are adulterated, usually by adding synthetic fragrances or a cheaper essential oil with a similar fragrance. This is especially true of the more expensive oils, such as rose, or those in high demand, like French lavender.

The best way to guarantee you are using good quality oils is to purchase from a reputable supplier who is also a trained aromatherapist, can tell you where the plant was grown and how it was distilled, and guarantee botanical purity. In the Appendix you'll find a list of recommended suppliers.

Hydrosols

Hydrosol (also called hydrolat) is the water part of the essential oil distillation process. After the bulk of the essential oil is removed, the water that is left behind contains the gentler, water soluble plant molecules and small traces of essential oil. This is hydrosol.

Hydrosols expand the range of things you can do with aromatics, because they are gentler than essential oils. You can replace any essential oil with its hydrosol equivalent for sensitive or vulnerable dogs. You can also use hydrosols in delicate areas where essential oils are too harsh. For example, around the eyes.

Hydrosols are easily digested, so are a much better option than essential oils for digestive problems and internal use. I also use them for deep-rooted emotional problems.

Unlike essential oils, hydrosols dissolve in water. You can put a few drops in a bowl of water and let your dog sniff or drink it whenever he likes. You can leave a calming hydrosol for him if he gets anxious when you go out. Or a little ginger hydrosol to help ease the discomfort of arthritis. You can also use this method to help dogs who don't want to interact with humans, as you can add the hydrosol to a bowl of water, then leave the area.

You can use the hydrosol instead of the more costly essential oils, such as rose (*Rosa damascena*); or those that are skin irritants, like clove (*Syzygium aromaticum*). There are also some plants that do not produce enough essential oil to collect, but are distilled only for the hydrosol. For example, witch hazel (*Hamamelis virginiana*), a hydrosol I use often for first aid.

Hydrosols require the same careful distillation process as essential oils. It is generally accepted that the best hydrosols are the first 30% of the distillation. Collecting more than that dilutes the active constituents. The purity of the water used also affects the end product.

Some people distill plants solely for the water (hydrosol). The essential oil is not removed. Strictly speaking, this is called aromatic water, not hydrosol. Aromatic water contains higher levels of essential oil so is slightly less gentle than a hydrosol.

Vegetable and herbal oils

Essential oils usually need to be diluted before use. For this we most commonly use vegetable and herbal oils, which is why they are also called carrier or base oils.

Vegetable oils are mostly extracted from the nuts, seeds or kernels of plants. Some of them, such as hemp or neem, are therapeutic in their own right. Others have little or no inherent fragrance or therapeutic action and make a perfect, neutral carrier oil for essential oils, especially for emotional/behavioral problems. If you have only one vegetable oil in your kit, opt for cold-pressed sunflower or jojoba.

Herbal oil, also known as macerated or infused oil, is made by soaking herbs in a cold-pressed vegetable oil, such as sunflower. Lipid (fat) soluble molecules are drawn out of the plant into the oil. These herbal oils are true aromatic extracts with powerful healing qualities.

Because essential oils don't contain the heavier lipid-soluble molecules, diluting them in macerated herbal oils is like putting the plant back together. This creates a unique healing synergy.

Herbal oils can also be used without essential oils in the long term care of conditions such as arthritis, or for wound care. Some vegetable oils, for example hemp or coconut, are good food supplements.

Good quality vegetable oils are not heated at any point in the production process, so always use traditional cold-pressed oil. Since pesticides and other chemical residues are easily carried over in the extraction process, choose organic whenever possible. Do not use the highly processed vegetable oils you find in supermarkets.

Macerated oils should be made using cold-pressed oils and pesticide free herbs.

That's a very brief summary of the aromatic extracts we will be using. Now, a little about the methodology.

THE METHOD

The system you will learn in this book is based on allowing your dogs to self-select the aromatics they need (zoopharmacognosy). Also, for best results when using aromatics, it is important to look at health holistically and understand stress. Let's explore these concepts a little....

Zoopharmacognosy

(Zoo = animal, pharma = medicine, cognosy = knowledge)

Zoopharmacognosy is a very long word for animal self medication. This scientific discipline studies an animal's instinctive drive to seek out the healing herbs and minerals he or she needs.

Animals are said to be self medicating when they eat something that is not a normal part of their diet. This can be a plant, fungi, soil or clay.

The most common example is dogs eating grass to cleanse their digestive tracts, clean their teeth and control worms. Observe carefully when your dog eats grass, and you will see that he is selecting his grasses very carefully.

More exotic examples are: monkeys eating bitter herbs to cleanse parasites; macaques rubbing aromatic plants into their fur to prevent fleas and heal skin sores; birds using insect repellent plants to line their nests; and elephants using clay as plasters for wounds. There are many more examples being observed as scientists study the phenomenon.

Scientists assume that animals find substances tasty if their bodies need a particular healing compound. When the body is healed, the plant is no longer tasty.

Self-selection

Domestic dogs retain the innate ability to select plant medicines. Such a useful biological survival mechanism is not easily lost, and evolutionarily speaking dogs have not been domesticated all that long. We use this instinctive ability and let dogs choose their own aromatics.

In the 20 years I have been working with animals and aromatics, self-selection has proved itself to be a safe, effective and powerful healing method that has many advantages. Not the least of which is that dogs love it.

The holistic view

You may have had the frustrating experience of multiple vet visits for the same problem. And each time the prescription is changed. For a while there might be even some improvement in the condition. But soon you are back to square one: itchy skin, fungal ears, or whatever problem brought you to the vet in the first place.

Maybe you got rid of the itching, but are soon back trying to get on top of Irritable Bowel Syndrome (IBS). This happens because modern medicine treats disease symptoms, not their causes.

The holistic view sees body, mind, emotions and environment, as one unit. With this view in mind we see that both problems arise from the same underlying imbalance.

In an holistic approach symptoms are clues we use to detect where the system has broken down.

Our aim is to rebalance your dog's whole system so he can heal himself. To do this we identify stressors and remove them, then support the self healing mechanism with natural medicines.

The aromatics your dog chooses can help you understand the whole condition. For instance, itching can be caused by diet, stress, or pain. Yarrow (*Achillea millefolium*) calms skin and is anti-inflammatory. Roman chamomile (*Anthemis nobilis*) calms skin and nervous stress. Spearmint (*Mentha Spicata*) stimulates digestion and is cooling. The oil your dog chooses provides clues to underlying problems and what else you can do to help.

For a full and lasting cure you must look at all the manifestations of dis-ease and create a healthy environment.

Stress & Wellness

Stress is the prime cause of dis-ease for animals. To have a truly healthy dog you must reduce stresses wherever possible. Stress can be defined as "anything that makes animals uncomfortable". *Dis*tress is when the system breaks down due to stress overload.

Not all stress is bad. Even chasing sticks provokes stress. As the chase/hunt switches are turned on adrenalin levels are raised. Joints and muscles are stressed by running, turning and stopping. But as long as there are no underlying problems, this is not distress. Too many stresses, or chronic stress, are what leads to distress, opening the door for disease.

Aromatics can help dogs cope with the everyday stresses of normal life. Such as family changes, moving home, or exposure to viruses. However, for best results be aware of what stresses dogs, and your dog in particular, and keep them to a minimum.

One of the major causes of stress for any animal is lack of self determination. We love our dogs, but our concern for their well-being often means we restrict their freedom and limit their choices.

You can't let your dog freely wander the streets, but you *can* let him participate in his own health care. Letting your dog self-select aromatic extracts reduces stress and improves health. Stress reduction plus essential oils is a powerful healing combination.

Other major causes of stress for modern dogs are:
- Inappropriate diet: dogs should eat a meat based diet.
- Over vaccination
- Chemical flea treatments
- Miscommunication with his person
- Unrealistic expectations about their behavior
- Lack of stimulation
- Over stimulation.

How to Use
Aromatic Extracts...

To Keep Your Dog Healthy

A romatics reduce stress and increase immune response, so are the perfect way to keep dogs healthy. I offer them to all my animals on a regular basis.

If I feel one of my fur friends is not quite as vital as usual, I let them sniff through my collection of oils and select the ones they want. I also do this when they are exposed to stressors, such as a change in routine or family composition.

Once they have selected their essential oil and carrier oil I dilute 1 drop of essential oil to 5 ml/1 tsp carrier and offer again.

Usually, they will have a small sniff, perhaps a little lick, and very quickly be back to their usual bouncy selves. Using this system regularly helps keep my dogs healthy and stop illness developing.

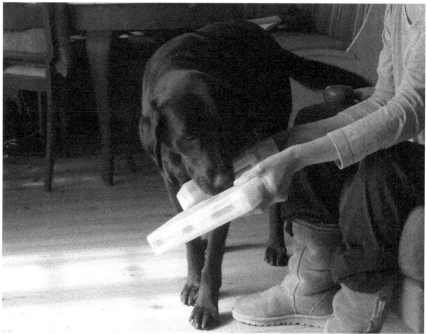

Here, Thor indicates the box that holds the oil he needs.

To Relieve A Specific Problem

If you offer aromatics on a regular basis, you reduce the chances of problems developing. Nevertheless, however well we care for our animals, sometimes things go wrong. When I address specific issues I make a short list of the essential oils and hydrosols that are most likely to help. I then let dogs choose between the aromatics on my shortlist.

I always use this method when a new animal joins the family to make sure he starts life with us in good health and clear of past traumas. Here's how to do it, step by step.

Make your shortlist

Think carefully about what you aim to achieve. Also consider your dog's character and any other problems he either has or had in the past. Thinking of all these things will help you choose the best remedy.

Don't just look at essential oils for the present symptoms, remember they are just a clue to the underlying imbalance. To clear the root cause, look for the aromatics that match the whole picture, past and present, physical and emotional.

The more you clarify your aims, the easier it will be to select the aromatics. If you say, "I want to make my dog feel better", you will have endless possibilities. When you look at the whole picture and include all physical, emotional and behavioral factors you narrow your choices.

So, "I want to help my dog's stiffness, he also seems to be more fearful since we moved house, and his coat is thin and dandruffy," is a much clearer goal.

Once you have set your goal, look at the list of <u>Aromatics for Specific Conditions</u> and check which aromatics are suggested for:

- Stiffness and/or pain,
- Fear,
- Confidence,
- Dandruff.

Sometimes you will find one essential oil that covers all your goals. Other times it will take two or three different oils to cover everything.

Next, look at the <u>Aromatic Cross Reference Chart</u> and see which of the possible oils/hydrosols most closely match your dog's issues. The more conditions that match your dog in each box, the more likely it is to be the best oil for the job.

Depending on the aromatics you have available, you can use essential oils and/or hydrosols. If you have both the essential oil and hydrosol offer both. He will indicate if he prefers the essential oil or the hydrosol.

Aim to have a short list of 3-5 essential oils/hydrosols. Your dog will probably select one or two.

Here is my shortlist for our example:

- Cedarwood (*Cedrus Atlantica*) for stiffness, circulation stimulant, fear, grounding after moving house, dandruff

- Angelica root (*Angelica archangelica*) circulation stimulant, to feel protected (fear)
- Geranium (*Pelargonium graveolens*) for scurfy skin, lack of confidence, moving home
- Yarrow (*Achillea millefolium*) protective, anti-inflammatory, fearful aggression

Let your dog smell each of the oils on your shortlist, one by one. With the **lid on**, pass the bottle under his nose quickly and gauge his response. He will move towards the ones he likes with his nose, maybe lick his lip a little. If he doesn't want the oil he will walk away or turn his head away.

Dilute the ones he selected and offer them again. This time let him interact with the oil/hydrosol however he choses.

Why to dilute?

I always dilute essential oils when using them with dogs, because they are potent. A tiny amount has strong effects, so there is no reason to use undiluted oils. Just as with aspirins, you don't use five when one will do the trick.

What's more, aromatics work better when diluted. Their molecules "curl up" when they are too densely packed, and stretch out to look for each other when in low concentration. Diluted essential oils are more easily absorbed by the body, so no energy is wasted on excretion, and you reduce the possibility of irritation or sensitization.

But the main reason I dilute is because the dogs have shown me they prefer it that way. I have seen dogs, who have been previously traumatized by smelling undiluted essential oils, run out of the room at the sight of one of those evil little glass bottles. The more sensitive the dog, the more important it is to dilute well.

Before we leave this question, open a bottle of essential oil and smell it. Now imagine that smell 100,000 time more powerfully! Do you feel overwhelmed at the thought? Well, a dog's sense of smell is at least that much more sensitive than yours, it could be as much as 1,000,000 times more so....

How to dilute essential oils

Essential oils should be diluted in a carrier oil. Pour the carrier oil into a small bottle. A five or ten milliliter glass bottle works best, available from most aromatherapy suppliers. The bottle should have a screw on cap, to keep the diluted oil fresh.

Label the bottle with the names of the essential oil and carrier oil and the dilution level. Wrap a piece of clear sticky tape around the label so that, when oily, it doesn't slip off. If stored in a cool dark place, the diluted oil will stay fresh for about 3 months,.

Dilute each essential oil/hydrosol separately. Do not blend. Your dog needs the freedom to interact individually with each extract. If you mix the oils, your dog is likely to refuse the blend when he goes off only one of the oils. Or, if he is really desperate, he may continue to take the blend just for the one oil he needs, increasing the risk of sensitization or irritation.

Rates of dilution, essential oil

Physical problems 1-3 drops of essential oil in 5 ml/1 tsp of carrier oil

Emotional problems/trauma 1-2 drops essential oil in 10 ml/2 tsp of carrier oil, or use hydrosol.

The more sensitive or delicate the dog, the higher the dilution should be (less essential oil more carrier). For puppies and the nervous or highly strung, use only hydrosols.

How to dilute hydrosols

You can use hydrosols undiluted for acute conditions, if your dog chooses to lick them. You do not need to dilute for washing wounds or soothing skin. However for long term use or sensitive dogs dilution is necessary. The general rule is for emotional problems (sensitive issues) and sensitive dogs dilute more.

You can start with as little as 1 drop in 1 cup/250ml of water. If your dog shows no interest in this dilution add more drops until he comes closer. If he leaves when you add more drops, just leave the water on the floor. Your dog will come back to it when the hydrosol has evaporated a little and the smell fades to a comfortable level.

If you have a strong, robust dog (not necessarily large in size, it could be a Jack Russell, we are talking robust character here) start with 1 teaspoon/5ml in 1 cup/250 ml. You have a lot of leeway with hydrosols, they are extremely safe. It is just a matter of finding your dog's comfort level.

Rates of dilution, hydrosols
Physical problems, start at 10% to 50% hydrosol in filtered water.
Emotional problems, 1-10 drops in 1 cup/250 ml of filtered water.

How to understand your dog's responses
Once you have diluted the aromatics your dog selected, offer them to him again. You must be patient when offering and watch carefully.

The key to using aromatics is understanding what your dog is saying when he responds to them. A dog's response can be so subtle you think nothing is happening. Or he may want to eat the bottle out of your hand. This depends on your dog's character and the nature of his imbalance.

When working with a dog on a particular problem, set yourself up for success. Make this quality one on one time with your dog, a quiet healing time for you to share together. Choose a time when there are no other distractions or excitements, such as food time or walks. Exclude other animals if they will be a distraction.

There are three major ways dogs choose to interact with aromatic extracts....

Inhalation
Your dog may just smell the oil, lying down quietly. He will go into a trance-like state, head lowered, eyes flickering as he processes what's happening. It may look like he is just lying there doing nothing. But if you observe carefully, you will see the eyes flickering and nostrils slightly flaring. If you move the bottle away, he may either follow the aroma with his nose, or glance at you quickly.

If there is no reaction when you move the bottle, replace the lid and wait for your dog to return from his relaxed space before offering another oil. Do not hurry the process and do not try to offer other oils until he has "come back", this may take half an hour or so. You can leave him to it.

I consider inhalation the most powerful way to deliver essential oils, since they go straight into the brain via the olfactory system. The brain then sends messages to the endocrine system, which trigger the appropriate responses in the body. That is why just smelling an essential oil can be enough to reduce pain, balance hormones, relieve itching, etc.

Oral

If your dog tries to lick or bite the bottle, dab a small amount of diluted oil on your hand, and allow him to lick it off. Repeat this three or four times in a session.

The sense of smell and taste function together, and most essential oils taken into the mouth will be absorbed into the olfactory cavity. Some of the oil will be absorbed into the blood system via mucous membranes, but only a minimal amount will reach the digestive system. Dogs are more likely to want to lick the oils if they have a physical problem or one that is not very deeply rooted.

Topical

Your dog may occasionally indicate a particular spot on his body by putting his nose to it, scratching, moving into you with his body, or communicating what he wants is some uniques way of his own. Often he is indicating an acupressure point, or a spot that is painful.

In this case, slowly move your hand into the area, allowing your dog to guide you to the exact spot, or to move away if he does not want oil on his body after all. Massage the area lightly until he moves away.

Level of interest

Your dog will interact differently with each essential oil at different times. In the beginning he may be intensely interested in one essential oil and less interested in others. But this interest can vary from day to day. As treatment progresses your dog should lose interest in all the oils.

Interest levels are classed as "keen", "moderate", or "none". Signs of keen interest are intense concentration on the bottle, trance, and/or eye flickering.

When the interest is moderate the dog will be easily distracted from the bottle, not go fully into trance, lick a little, then sniff around. I offer the remedy twice a day when interest is keen, once a day when moderate.

Dogs will normally start to lose interest in the oils within three days to a week of the first session. In rare cases your dog will lose interest after one session, especially if the problem was not deep seated. By the time your dog loses interest in the oil completely you will normally see a significant reduction of the problem.

The Illustrated "How to"

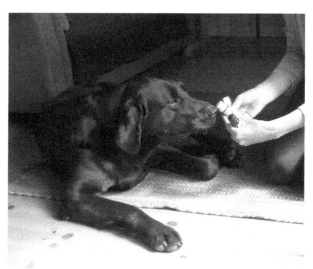

1.Let him smell the oils on your shortlist, with the bottle caps on.

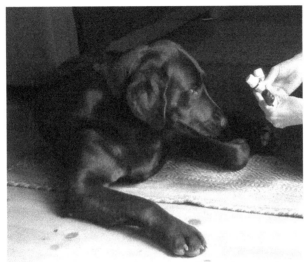

2. Thor pulls his nose away from the middle oil, so I take it away.

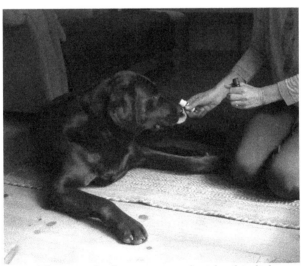

3. Thor says 'yes' to carrot seed with a big lick.

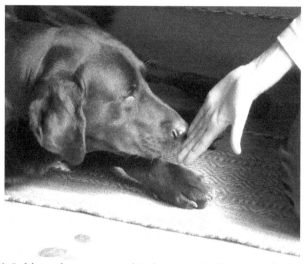

4. I dilute the carrot seed 2 drops in 5ml/1 tsp sunflower and put it on my hand for Thor to sniff or lick as he chooses.

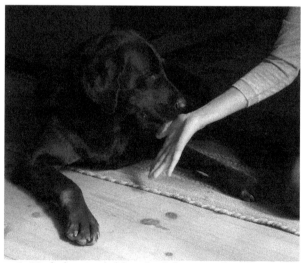

5. He licks ½ ml diluted oil from my hand twice, cleaning up thoroughly each time.

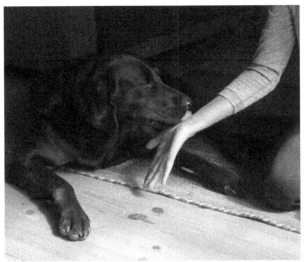

6. The third time I add oil to my hand he licks my wrist, avoiding the oil. This means he has had enough internally but is still taking it by olfaction.

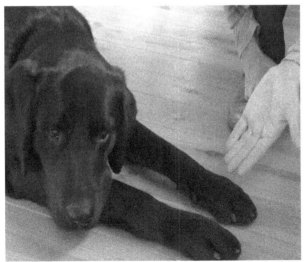

7. The second diluted essential oil, lavender, he just inhales. This is a typical pose for a dog when inhaling and slipping into trance.

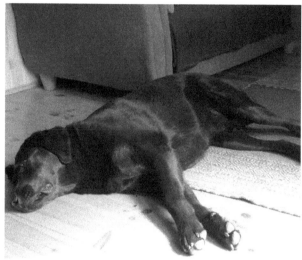

8. He then lies down, but before he does so he licks his tummy.
I think he may want a little of the lavender rubbed there.

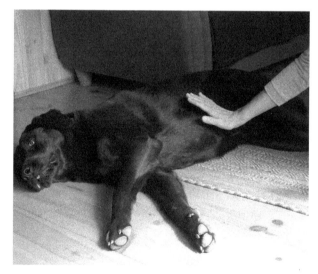

9. I hold my oily hand just above the spot
he was licking, he doesn't move.

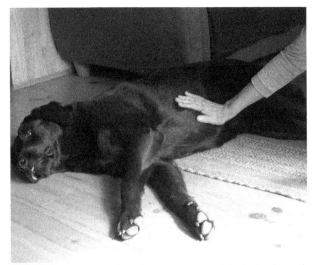

10. So I put my hand on his tummy and hold it there for
a minute or two, until he sighs.

For Environmental Control

Essential oils are volatile, meaning they disperse easily into the air. An easy and natural way to use them is to diffuse them. Do this in an area where your dog can choose to hang out or leave. You can use an electric diffuser, an aromatherapy stone, or just put a drop or two of essential oil on a tissue and leave it in a warm spot, out of your dog's reach. You can also put a few drops of hydrosol in a dish of water for a similar but gentler effect.

Limit infectious disease

Diffusing is particularly useful if you want to limit the spread of viruses, such as in a kennel or rescue shelter. *Eucalyptus radiata* and bergamot (*Citrus bergamia*) work well together for this. But many essential oils are immune stimulant, respiratory disinfectant and/or limit airborne bacteria, so you are spoilt for choice. See which ones your dog prefers.

Calm training classes

You can also diffuse essential oils in group situations such as dog training classes, where you might want to encourage calmness or focus. You can allow dogs to be as close to or far from the diffuser as suits them.

You can put frankincense in a burner or diffuser to help dogs who are scared of fireworks or thunder.

Allow your dog freedom of movement when diffusing. Do not shut him up in the room, he still needs to be able to choose to interact.

Diffusion works well for:

- Fears and phobias, such as fireworks
- Separation anxiety and other mental stress
- Preventing airborne bacteria and the spread of disease
- Inter-pack tension

FOR BUG CONTROL

Natural resistance

Healthy dogs, fed fresh whole food, are more able to resist bugs. By contrast, poor diet, high stress levels, flea treatments and vaccines all lower immunity and make infestation and irritation more likely. Regularly offering essential oils makes sure the immune system is in tip-top shape, ready to repel bugs and the diseases they often carry.

Make your own natural repellent

But in some climates and some seasons bugs can get the best of even the healthiest dogs. Then aromatics are your best ally in the fight against fleas, ticks and mosquitoes, because you can make your own 100% natural repellents.

Bug repellents made specifically for your dog, with his help, are more effective than anything shop bought. What's more, they have no unpleasant side effects and boost the immune system instead of lowering it. Plus, they are really fun to make!

My most tried and true bug control method is to mix essential oils and neem oil in a hydrosol gel. Neem oil is one of nature's strongest insecticides. Since the smell can be unpleasant, or even offensive to some people, you definitely need to dilute well. But it really works and has been tested to bee effective at 1% dilution (1 ml in 100 ml/ 1 tablespoon in a cup).

I use sweet smelling insect repellent essential oils to help mask the neem smell. Geranium, lemongrass and patchouli are some of my favorites. But, again, each dog has his own preference and many essential oils repel bugs, so I offer a selection of essential oils and hydrosols and let him choose.

A downside to using essential oils as bug repellents is that they evaporate quickly, so don't last very long. Neem oil lingers, and hydrosols do a good job of coating the skin/hair for longer lasting effects.

Here's how to do it:

Combine in a bowl
- 50 ml aloe vera gel
- 5 ml neem oil
- 3 drops cedarwood essential oil
- 3 drops lavender essential oil
- 3 drops lemongrass essential oil

The final gel should be the consistency of hair conditioner, so slowly stir in up to,

- 50 ml geranium hydrosol

Rub a small amount through the coat every few days. Concentrate on the places bugs travel, the ruff, between the legs and around the ears. Reapply if you know you are going to a bug infested area or after swimming.

More Aromatic Bug Repellents
- A kerchief soaked in bug repellent gel and tied around your dog's neck. This is good if you are going to a heavily infested area, such as a walk in the woods of Wisconsin.

- A few drops of lemongrass hydrosol in a bowl of water for your dog to drink. This inhibits fleas

- You can add a few squirts of the above lotion to ¼ bucket of water as a coat conditioning/flea repelling wash. Wet your dog down first then sponge on from the bucket, as much as possible leave to air dry. This is a good system in summer when it's hot and you can leave them out in the garden to dry.

- Hydrosol spray, safer for daily applications if you feel it is needed, or around the face to protect from mosquitoes. Dilute hydrosol such as eucalyptus or lavender (or both) with distilled water 50/50.

- Another very effective method is to mix ½ cup diatomaceous earth (food grade), ¼ cup neem leaf powder, and ¼ cup kaolin clay, add a drop or two of cedarwood or lavender, and store in a plastic squeeze bottle. Dust underbelly and ruff lightly, once a week, or as required.

As First Aid

Essential oils for traumatic injury

Hydrosols and essential oils can deal with pretty much all your first aid needs, such as stings, scratches, bumps and bruises. Undiluted hydrosols can be used to wash wounds, heal bruises and relieve pain, or made into gels to speed healing. Essential oils can be antiseptic, anti-bacterial, anti-inflammatory, relieve pain and aid healthy skin repair.

I also use essential oils in true first response situations, such as traumatic injury, while waiting for the vet. I offer neroli (*Citrus aurantium var bigarade*) for shock, helichrysum (*Helichrysum italicum*) for impact injuries, and yarrow (*Achillea millefolium*) to stop bleeding and relieve trauma. You could also use lavender (*Lavandula officinalis)* to do any of those things, but it is not quite as powerful. Offering aromatics while waiting for the vet will reduce stress and help speed recovery.

For healing minor injuries I combine essential oils, hydrosols and herbal oils, offering essential oils for inhalation and making a topical gel as well.

Co-operative health care

When healing injuries I still let my dogs guide me, even though this is when I am most tempted to force them to take something — anything! — to relieve my worry. Experience and some very wise dogs have taught me better.

If I need to wash a wound I offer a choice of hydrosol, such as lavender, helichrysum or witch hazel. Then let them choose between clay or gel to protect it. I usually have a first aid gel and clay ready for use. But if I didn't I would allow them to select the essential oils to add to the gel as well.

In this situation I am asking the dog, "Do you strongly object to me using this?". I will not force topical application if my dog resists, but I am not looking for engagement on a deep level, just acceptance.

This may seem extreme to you, but the truth is when dogs are first injured they will generally accept help. As healing progresses they will start to refuse. The body heals itself, given the right conditions, and your dog knows if/when help is needed.

Aromatics rebalance the whole system as well as working directly on wounds, so you can apply them less frequently than a standard antibiotic application. And the really wonderful thing in a first aid situation is, when you have the right oil for the occasion your dogs don't resist being treated. No more struggling to dress a wound, that's one stress out of the window already!

Essential first aid kit

Hydrosols are great for washing wounds and to poultice injuries. You can also replace any essential oil with its hydrosol equivalent.

Hydrosols
- Witch hazel: mild disinfectant, stops bruising, soothes skin, astringent
- Thyme ct thymol or Tea tree (*Melaleuca alternifolia*) disinfectant
- Cornflower: soothing, eye wash

Carrier oils

- Aloe vera gel: anti-inflammatory, skin soothing
- Calendula oil: anti-inflammatory, wound healing, anti-fungal, soothing

Essential oils

- Helichrysum: antiseptic, anti-bruising, anti-inflammatory
- Lavender: antiseptic, wound healing, prevents scarring and proud flesh
- Neroli: for shock
- Plai: anti-inflammatory, analgesic
- Valerian: sedative
- Yarrow: stops bleeding, disinfectant, creates a protective barrier over the wound, anti-inflammatory, releases trauma.

I always have a couple of home made gels ready in my first aid kit, such as those in the section below. They are a great way to soothe minor irritations and wounds.

How To Make
Aromatic Lotions

When to use topicals

I don't use topical application very often. Why? Because healing happens from the inside out.

Skin problems are often the first place that the body lets us know it is out of balance. The skin is the largest organ and the safest place for the body to clear toxins. When offering aromatics to re-balance the immune or digestion system, problems such as itchy skin usually clear by themselves.

However, there are some situations that call for external application to help speed recovery and relieve irritation. Or to inhibit secondary bacterial infection, as in lickomas.

Anytime an imbalance manifests in the skin you can add the essential oil or hydrosol your dog chooses to a gel, as well has offering them individually.

Why we use gels

I use a water based gel as the carrier for topical applications. I never use oil based lotions or creams when working with dogs. Apart from the fact that a dog covered in oily lotions is going to play havoc with your carpets, water based gels are easier to make at home.

Another advantage of a water based gel is that essential oils avoid water and are drawn to lipids (fat). So they move quickly out of the gel and into the dog's skin. Sooner or later dogs will want to lick themselves clean. If you use a water based gel, the essential oil will already have been absorbed into the skin by the time he gets around to cleaning himself.

These gels are non-toxic and it will not harm your dog to lick them. But you want them to stay on the skin long enough to do their job. Interestingly, dogs do not usually lick the gel right off when the right remedy is applied. If your dog does try to lick straight away, you can offer him the bottle of gel to smell, or let him lick a little of the gel from your hand while the gel absorbs.

How to use gels

The first step to making a gel is to allow your dog to approve of the essential oils you have chosen. For example, if you are making a wound gel, you could offer helichrysum, lavender, yarrow and rosalina. Take the 2 or 3 he shows the most interest in and add them to the gel. Add more drops of the oils he liked best, less of the others. So you might end up with 3 drops of rosalina, 2 of helichrysum and 1 of yarrow in 30 ml/2 tablespoons of gel.

Before application

Once you have concocted the gel, let your dog smell it again, and then apply to affected areas. He will show you exactly where he needs it by moving into your hand or moving away. If he doesn't like the smell, it may be too strong. Add another teaspoon of gel or plain water.

Offer your dog the gel to smell before each application, and listen to where he wants it applied. If he wants to, you can also let him lick some from your hand. As the problem clears he will want it applied less frequently.

He may decide he doesn't want the gel any more when you think he still needs it. In this case, offer different oils for selection, and adjust the gel. If he shows no interest in any of the oils, the healing is going well and he doesn't need any more help. Trust him!

QUICK GEL RECIPE

Measurement converter: 100ml = almost ½ cup
250ml=1 cup
5ml = 1 teaspoon
15 ml = 1 tablespoon

This recipe uses store bought aloe vera gel, such as you find in health food stores. Look for a gel that is fragrance free and as free of additives as possible (nothing store bought will be absolutely pure).

To make 100 ml of lotion or 250 ml of spray.

Ingredients:

- 50 ml aloe gel,
- 5 ml of herbal oil (optional)
- A maximum total of 20 drops essential oils, maximum 3 essential oils in one blend
- 100-250 ml of distilled water or hydrosol, as required

Procedure:

Put the gel in a glass bowl.

Pour the vegetable oil into a stainless steel measuring spoon and add your chosen essential oils.

Mix oils into the gel with a glass stirring rod, or stainless steel whisk, or wooden chopstick.

Slowly whisk in water or hydrosol to thin the gel to your desired consistency.

For wounds and itchy skin: The gel can be fairly thick, like a rich body lotion. A drop of gel should sit on your hands without spreading.

To make a spray: Keep adding water or hydrosol until the mix is thin enough to spray.

You can adapt this basic gel to every situation by changing the essential oils, hydrosols and herbal oils you use.

HYDROSOL GEL

A slightly more advanced version is to make your own gel. This way you ensure that your potion is 100% natural. You could also use distilled water, or aloe juice for the liquid part of the gel. But I like to make up a gel using hydrosols. When you add essential oils and herbal oils you make a powerful healing potion. Or you could leave out the essential oils to treat puppies or other sensitives.

Ingredients:

100 ml hydrosol of your choice,

1 teaspoon xanthan or guar gum (available in some health food stores and many aromatherapy suppliers)

Procedure:

Use either a hand mixer or blender to make the gel.

First warm the bowl or blender with boiling water. This sterilizes the container and makes the hydrosol gel more easily.

Pour hydrosol into the warmed bowl/blender.

Sprinkle the xanthan gum on top of the hydrosol.

Whisk for about 5 minutes or until the xanthan gum has completely dissolved and the gel has thickened.

The gel should be thick enough to hold its shape in your hand without spreading when dropped from a teaspoon. In any of the following recipes you can use an appropriate hydrosol gel instead of aloe vera gel.

A FEW RECIPES

Here are some examples of gels for common problems. But don't let these limit you. Follow the principle of setting your goal and letting your dog select the aromatics he wants, and you are sure to come up with great combinations of your own.

One hint, when making potions, the final smell should make you go, "Aaah!", when you smell it. Even if the fragrance is not something you would wear on a date, the ingredients should blend harmoniously without any one smell dominating. Play around, have fun, be creative!

Disinfectant wound gel

- 50 ml aloe vera gel
- 5 drops helichrysum essential oil
- 2 drops lavender essential oil
- 3 drops yarrow essential oil
- 20 ml thyme hydrosol (or as much as you need to thin the gel)

Wash the wound with disinfectant hydrosol, such as tea tree or thyme. Then apply a dab of gel with a clean finger or cotton bud.

Scar reducing wound gel

- 50 ml lavender hydrosol gel
- 5 ml calendula
- 3 drops helichrysum essential oil
- 2 drops frankincense essential oil

You can encourage healthy skin repair with this gel once the wound has started to heal. Apply once or twice a day to begin with, or as your dog guides you.

Anti-inflammatory pain gel

- 50 ml aloe vera gel
- 5 ml hypericum oil
- 7 drops plai
- 5 drops juniper berry
- 3 drops yarrow
- 50 ml peppermint hydrosol

Apply as needed or when and where your dog guides you. My old girl would go and stand beside the shelf where I kept the bottle when she was feeling stiff and achy.

Lickomas

For best results, trace and remove the underlying cause of the lickoma. It is not necessarily a skin problem. A dog may lick himself raw because of pain in the neck or spinal column. Or, digestive discomfort. Or stress. While you work to alleviate the cause, this gel will help prevent secondary infection and speed healing of the sore.

- 15 ml thyme hydrosol gel
- 5 ml comfrey or calendula herbal oil
- 2 drops Lavender essential oil
- 1 drop helichrysum
- 1 drop rosalina

Ear wash

If your dog gets "gunky ears", stick to a grain free diet and reduce stress to strengthen the immune system. Don't use essential oils inside the ear.

- 15 ml thyme hydrosol gel
- 15 ml witch-hazel hydrosol
- 5 ml calendula herbal oil

Mix together. Soak a cotton ball with gel, wipe out ear thoroughly.

Dental Care

The best way to prevent dental disease is to feed raw meaty bones, appropriate to your dog's size. Feeding home-cooked or raw diets are also much less likely to create an unhealthy build up of periodontal bacteria. A raw fed dog is also unlikely to have bad breath. If you do need to brush your dog's teeth, don't use essential oils. The most effective and safe natural toothpaste is:

Tooth Powder

- 30 grams bentonite clay
- 5 grams green clay

- 5 grams turmeric, or cinnamon powder (whichever your dog prefers, let him smell and decide)
- An optional 5 grams neem leaf powder, if your dog likes the smell
- 5 grams baking soda
- A pinch of salt.

Dampen a toothbrush or finger and rub the powder into the gums, et voila!

Tooth clay

For cases of serious dental decay you can make a clay mask.

- 15 grams green French clay
- 15 grams witch-hazel or tea tree hydrosol (or as needed)
- 10 ml coconut oil (soften if necessary)

Combine all ingredients, mixing well until they are a soft paste. Smear liberally on gums.

Odor control

I am often asked for "dog perfume". No, not a fragrance to make you smell of dog—although your furry friend would probably prefer that—something to make dogs smell less doggy and more like us.

An unpleasant doggy smell is usually the result of a stressful lifestyle. "Dog breath" is a direct result of what you feed them. Healthy dogs smell good.

The first step to an odor free dog is feeding fresh whole food and keeping stresses to a minimum. Using essential oils to keep them healthy, and making your own flea gels, will also improve the smell.

But if your dog just got "skunked", or rolled in something stinky, wash well with a natural olive or neem oil bar soap and then use hydrosols as a rinse or spray. But let your dog choose the hydrosols he prefers.

As a rule, the sweeter hydrosols, such as geranium, mask smell best. Add a teaspoon of apple cider vinegar to help neutralize odors.

SAFE USAGE

Aromatics are a safe option for animal health IF we use them as nature intended: short term and well-diluted. Combine that with zoopharmacognosy (animal self-selection) and you can't go wrong. However, here are a few more specific safety points.

The most common problem

Anything can cause harm when over used. The most common problem in the world of aromatherapy is when long term exposure to essential oils causes an allergic reaction. This is known as sensitization. This usually comes about through over use of topical applications. But shutting animals up in a closed space while diffusing can also cause sensitization, or a toxic build up in the liver.

Changing nature

Although self-selection is based on natural processes, an essential oil or dried herb is not the same as the total plant in nature. We have removed much of its bulk and many of nature's own regulatory measures. Thus, it's important to dilute essential oils and regulate your dogs' intake accordingly.

Further, self-selection is based on taking something until you feel better. Sometimes the trigger for the "not good" feeling is something in the environment. For example, diet or other stresses. If you do not remove the source of the problem, your dog may not know when to stop. This increases the risk of sensitization.

Know when to call in the professionals

If your dog has disease symptoms, it is crucial to consult with a veterinarian or qualified natural health practitioner as soon as possible. While natural medicine is great for your home pharmacy, sometimes you need stronger medicine. Building a good relationship with your vet ensures that your dog has the best possible care. Together you can work out a treatment plan that includes aromatics.

Some basic guidelines for safety's sake

- Allow your dog to self-select

- Dilute your essential oils well

- Use high grade essential oils from a reputable supplier

- Allow your dog to smell EACH aroma before EACH application. To apply without offering is at best annoying (imagine being smothered in a perfume you hated with no way to wash it off) and at worst dangerous

- In the unlikely event of your dog showing a reaction, such as skin irritation or shortness of breath, immediately discontinue use and contact a vet

- Store essential oils in a cool, dark place with their caps firmly closed

- Never leave essential oil bottles in reach of dogs. They have been known to steal them from counter tops and swallow them

- Do not use on pregnant dogs without further guidance from a professional

- Pay attention to the cautions and safety issues with each essential oil

- If your dog is still interested in oils after 2 weeks, contact a professional for advice

- Avoid using wintergreen (*Gaultheria procumbens*), birch (*Betula lenta*), cinnamon (*Cinnamomum zeylanicum*), tea tree (*Melaleuca alternifolia*), oregano (*Origanum vulgare*) and other hot, mucous membrane irritant oils

- Finally, whatever you do, when you have a problem, don't go to the internet and canvas the opinions of well meaning but unqualified people. They have no special training in animal aromatherapy and do not specifically know your dog.

Losing control

The hardest thing about allowing dogs to self-select aromatics is letting go of the notion that YOU know best! We may think something is wrong and want to fix it with an essential oil. But in basically healthy dogs, most things get better with time and patience. And sometimes things that concern us or we think are problems are actually nature's way of healing.

A good example of this is a sore leg. When a dog limps, our conditioning says pain killer, and we may want to rub something onto the leg. But pain is nature's way of saying, "stop, rest, heal". If we take away the pain, we slow the body's own healing mechanisms. You might think that a pain relieving oil, such as plai may be helpful in this situation. But if your dog says "No thanks", please respect that. If you go ahead and apply the oil anyway, you are likely to cause distress and slow down healing.

Dogs are working under nature's guidance, in tune with their instincts and know exactly what is needed.

Your Aromatic Pharmacy

What you need to get started

Starting your aromatic collection can seem daunting and expensive at first. But it doesn't have to be. I suggest you start with 5 to 10 essential oils, 3 or 4 hydrosols, and a couple of base oils. But you could start with as few as 5 essential oils and 1 carrier oil. It depends on your pocket book and your animal family and what they need.

One way to start your collection is to buy the few essential oils or hydrosols you think your dog needs most. Then buy more as you need them, slowly building your collection, getting to know each item through hands-on experience and visible results.

Here is a list of aromatics that should cover most common eventualities. You can buy them as a kit through the Essential Animals website, or individually from your favorite supplier.

General Use Starter Kit
Essential oils:
Bergamot (Citrus bergamia)
Carrot seed (Daucus carota)
Cedarwood (Cedrus atlantica)
Frankincense (Boswellia carterii)
Lavender (Lavandula angustifolia)
Lemongrass (Cymbopogon citratus)
Roman chamomile (Anthemis nobilis)
Spearmint (Mentha spicata)
Yarrow (Achillea millefolium)
Vetiver (Vetiveria zizanoides)

Hydrosols:
Melissa (Melissa officinalis)
Neroli (Citrus aurantium var bigarade)
Witch hazel (Hamamelis virginiana)

Carrier oils
Sunflower (Helianthus anuus)
Calendula (Calendula officinalis)
Hemp (Cannabis sativa)
See the Appendix for suppliers in Europe and the US.

STORAGE

- Aromatics need to be stored in a cool dark, animal proof place (a fridge is best).

- Do not leave them on kitchen counters or suchlike, as dogs will go to great lengths to reach them when they need them.

- Keep aromatics away from direct sunlight and heat.

- All aromatics are best stored in glass bottles. Essential oils will destroy plastic containers.
- Hydrosols must be refrigerated.

Each item has its own shelf life, with some of the more delicate carrier oils starting to oxidize after 3 months (flaxseed). Some essential oils improve with age. As a general guide, the heavier, thicker essential oils, like vetiver, last longer. The lightweight citrus and pine essential oils last for a year. Check with your supplier for recommended shelf life on each item.

Whatever the label on the bottle says (European regulations require a 3 year "use by" date), shelf life is dictated by how you keep them. Essential oils oxidize with exposure to light and air, which makes them more likely to cause sensitization when put on the skin. It is best to buy smaller bottles more often, and make sure your supplier is also storing the oils properly.

Hydrosols have a low pH index, which inhibits bacterial growth. However, the pH level rises with age, along with the risk of bacterial contamination. The lower the pH the more stable the hydrosol, and the longer they will last.

To make your aromatics last longer, avoid introducing bacteria into the bottles. Don't put your fingers, or your dog's nose, on the top of an open bottle of hydrosol or carrier oil. Decant into smaller bottles for offering to keep the storage bottles clean.

Essential oil profiles

Angelica Root
(Angelica Archangelica)

History and Character

Angelica is a large, graceful plant that can grow to a height of 2 meters/6 ft. The whole plant exudes the energetic depth and reach, which mirrors angelica's healing power. Its roots go deep into the earth and strong tall stem—"reaching to the heavens"—supports a large white/green umbrella-like flower. The flower can be seen as protective, as well as open and receptive.

Angelica root oil has been traditionally used to protect against "the Plague", for nervous hysteria, as a general tonic, for "fortifying the spirit", and for female disorders. It strengthens the liver and steadies the heart. Angelica opens us to healing, reconnects us to our inner innocence and is said to "connect us to the angels". Angelica is innocent and strong at the same time and is very effective where fears or compulsive behavior have been triggered by a traumatic incident when very young.

Principal Uses

Physical

- Arthritis
- Chronic bronchial disorders
- Circulatory problems
- Cushing's syndrome and other metabolic disorders
- Dogs who have shut down due to chronic pain or stress
- Immune stimulant, especially for those run down by a long illness
- Liver dysfunction
- Loss of appetite, including anorexia

- Lymphatic problems
- Stress related digestive disorders

Behavioral

- Chronic anxiety
- Fears born out of early childhood traumas
- Strengthens the nerves, especially where there is hysteria brought on by nervous exhaustion

I most often use Angelica' for:

- Fear or compulsive behavior, especially after one or more traumatic incidents in early life
- Old dogs who are emotionally hardened or have chronic pain
- If dogs shows no interest in any of the other oils offered.

Extraction and Characteristics: Steam distilled from roots. The oil is a colorless liquid, which becomes slightly golden brown as it matures.

Fragrance: Sweet, sharp, pungent, with earthy undertones.

Actions: Antifungal, antispasmodic, antitoxic, antibacterial, carminative, digestive, diuretic, expectorant, febrifuge, general tonic, neurotonic.

Safety & Cautions: Non-toxic, non-irritant. Angelica root oil can be phototoxic when applied undiluted to skin. Avoid exposure to sun for 12 hours after application. Avoid use with diabetes.

Maximum dilution 2 drops in 5 ml/1 tsp.

Bergamot
(Citrus bergamia)

History and Character

Named for the city of Bergamo in northern Italy (Lombardy), this small tree (3.5 meters/12 ft. tall) resembles a miniature orange. Traditionally, it has been used for fever and worms. It is said to kill airborne bacteria and was used to stop the spread of infection in hospitals. One of the main qualities of bergamot is its balancing effect. This is particularly useful when things are out of control, as in growths, tumors and, on an emotional level, moods that swing between extremes. Bergamot's sharp, sweet smell is uplifting and clean, cutting through stagnant energies to release pent up emotions. It has a profound antidepressant effect, especially for those who turn anger and frustration in on themselves, as in self mutilation or obsessive compulsive behavior.

Principal Uses

Physical

- Brings bio-system into balance
- Genito-urinary tract infections
- Post parturition
- Ringworm
- Tumors, warts, growths of all kinds
- Viral infection

Behavioral

- Depression
- Frustrated irritability
- Snappiness

I most often use Bergamot for:

- Warts, growths and tumors, especially if the dog is snappy, intolerant or withdrawn.
- Changeable, moody individuals with unpredictable temperament.

Extraction and Characteristics: cold-pressed from the skin of the fruit. The oil is a clear green color.

Fragrance: A fresh, citrus aroma, with a slightly green edge.

Actions: Antibacterial, antiseptic, antispasmodic, antiviral, calmative, cicatrizant, febrifuge, parasiticide, sedative, stomachic, tonic, vermifuge.

Safety & cautions: Whole bergamot oil is phototoxic, so should not be applied to exposed skin up to 12 hours before exposure to ultra violet. Otherwise it is non-toxic and relatively non-irritant. While it is possible to buy bergapten-free bergamot, I never use it. Because when given the choice dogs consistently choose the whole oil over the altered one.

Maximum dilution 3 drops in 5 ml/1 tsp.

Cajeput
(Melaleuca Cajeputi Powell)

History and Character

Cajeput is native to Indonesia, Malaysia, Southeast Asia and tropical Australia. It is a tall evergreen tree with thick, pointed leaves and white flowers. Traditionally, it has been used for joint pains, earache, respiratory problems and for repelling head lice and fleas. Cajeput is also known as white tea tree and is from the same family as tea tree and rosalina. It shares the energetic sharpness and disinfectant properties of these oils. As with many of the Metal oils, cajeput focuses and cleanses energetic space. It can be useful in cutting through obsessive behavior by sharpening the mind and freeing it from a sense of entrapment.

Principal Uses

Physical

- Circulatory problems and arthritis
- Coughs and viral infections of the lungs
- Fleas
- General immune tonic
- Infected wounds

Behavioral

- Claustrophobia
- Obsessive compulsive behavior

I most often use Cajeput for:

Obsessive behavior, such as tail chasing, especially if dogs have breathing problems or a tendency toward lung infections.

Extraction and Characteristics: Steam distilled from the fresh leaves and twigs. The oil is a pale yellowy green liquid.

Fragrance: Camphoraceous, "medicinal"', with a slightly fruity edge.

Actions: Antirheumatic, antiseptic, antispasmodic, expectorant, febrifuge, insecticide, pulmonary disinfectant, tonic and stimulant.

Safety & cautions: Non-toxic, non-sensitizing but can irritate skin in high concentrations. For topical application dilute well. Avoid contact with mucous membranes.

Maximum dilution 3 drops in 5 ml/1 tsp.

Carrot seed
(Daucus carota)

History and Character

Wild carrot has a graceful, white flower growing from a succulent root. It is similar to the yellow carrot we know so well, but smaller and paler. The finest carrot seed essential oil is wild harvested in France, where the plant can be found in the fields and hedgerows of rural areas. The oil is well accepted by all types of dogs and is nourishing, both physically and emotionally. Carrot seed regenerates liver cells, helps repair damaged skin, rebuilds poor quality coats and nails, and encourages the production of healthy tissue in smooth muscles. This is the oil to use if there is any history of physical or emotional neglect, abandonment or starvation. Because of its connection to nourishment, it is a good oil for loss of appetite for food and life itself. Like a true earth mother, it responds to our needs and helps regenerate the system from the inside out.

Principal Uses

Physical

- Anorexia
- Flatulence
- Heart murmurs
- Liver damage
- Loss of appetite
- Malnutrition (past or present)
- Poor skin and nails
- Slow healing wounds
- Ulcers
- Worms

Behavioral

- Depression
- Emotional neglect or abandonment

- Loss of will to live

I most often use Carrot Seed for:

- Past or present, emotional or physical abandonment or neglect.

- An inability to give or receive nurture, especially if dogs are underweight, heal slowly or have poor quality coats or nails.

Extraction and Characteristics: Steam distilled from the dried seeds.

Fragrance: Damp earth, sweet, musty, warm.

Actions: Anthelmintic, antiseptic, carminative, detoxicant, diuretic, emmenagogue, hepatic, regenerative, smooth muscle relaxant, stimulant, tonic, vasodilator.

Safety & Cautions: Generally non-toxic, non-sensitizing. Can be harsh on skin and mucous membranes, dilute well.

Maximum dilution 3 drops in 5 ml/1 tsp.

Cedarwood Atlas
(Cedrus Atlantica)

History and Character

This magnificent tree is graceful and powerful with an awesome presence. It is native to the Atlas Mountains of Morocco and thought to be related to the Cedars of Lebanon. It is also closely related to the Himalayan cedar (*Cedrus Deodora*), which produces an essential oil that can be used interchangeably with the Atlas cedar.

Cedarwood has a long tradition of religious use in various cultures, as an incense and for building temples. The Egyptians used it for cosmetics and embalming. The cedar tree grows in the high mountains, where the air is clean and fresh. The tree has deep spreading roots and a tall straight trunk. The branches are flexible, moving in the wind but anchored to the central trunk.

Cedarwood oil grounds and centers us in our being, helping us to take a deep breath so we can face up to tough situations. It helps those who feel alienated, or fear that they don't have the strength to "hold it together", or generally feel overwhelmed by circumstances they have no control over.

Cedarwood gives inner calm in times of instability and is one of the oils to try if you are moving house or making similar major life changes.

Principal Uses

Physical

- Asthma
- Catarrh
- Hair loss
- Insect repellent
- Edema
- Weak kidneys or back
- Wheezing

Behavioral
- Fear, timidity
- Lack of willpower
- New home or moving house

I most often use Cedarwood for:
- Those who are unsettled by their surroundings or have just moved home.
- Timid fearful dogs, especially if there is a history of backache, kidney problems or hair loss.

Extraction and Characteristics: Steam distilled from wood, stumps and sawdust. It is a yellow, amber viscous oil.

Fragrance: A warm, woody, slightly camphoraceous odor.

Actions: Anticatarrhal, antiparasitic, antirheumatic, anti-seborrhea, cicatrizant, diuretic, expectorant, general tonic, lymphatic decongestant.

Safety & Cautions: Non-toxic and non-irritant in prescribed doses.

Maximum dilution 5 drops in 5 ml/1 tsp.

Chamomile, Roman
(Anthemis Nobilis, Chamamaelum Nobile)

History and Character

Roman Chamomile is a small, half spreading herb with feathery leaves and daisy like flowers. A sweet and gentle plant, delicate yet sturdy. Native to southern and western Europe, it is widely cultivated throughout Europe and the United States.

This pale blue oil, is similar to its cousin German chamomile, but less anti-inflammatory and more suited to those who are likely to make a fuss about every little thing, rather than "man up" and bear it stoically. Roman chamomile is ideal for those who are constitutionally nervous, "jumping out of their skins" and over reactive, especially if suffering from diarrhea when anxious.

The oil calms the nerves, stomach and skin, and helps them live more comfortably in their skins, physically and emotionally. For me it is "the child's oil", as it is gentle, soothing and works well for "growing up" problems, such as teething, colic and restlessness. It also helps dogs who are fearful or nervous with children and soothes immature tantrums and outbursts of emotion, however old you are.

Principal Uses

Physical
- Diarrhea
- Eczema
- Inflamed, itchy skin
- Nervous digestive problems
- Stress related skin problems
- Sweet itch

Behavioral
- Constitutional nervousness
- Fear, nervousness or intolerance of children
- Nervous aggression
- Restlessness

I most often use Roman Chamomile for:

- Nervous flighty dogs, especially if they suffer from itchy, irritable skin, or stress related upset stomachs.

- Any issues involving children, and frustration or angry outbursts.

Extraction and Characteristics: Steam distilled from the flower heads. A pale, blue, mobile liquid, that turns yellow with age.

Fragrance: Fruity, herbaceous, apple like, with a bitter note.

Actions: Analgesic, anti-inflammatory, anti-neuralgic, antiparasitic, antiseptic, antispasmodic, carminative, digestive, sedative, tonic vulnerary.

Safety & Cautions: Generally non-toxic and non-irritant. It can cause dermatitis in some individuals.

Maximum dilution 5 drops in 5 ml/1 tsp.

Clary Sage
(Salvia Sclarea)

History and Character

Clary Sage is a sturdy perennial herb with hairy, pale green, purple tinged leaves and insignificant blue flowers. Native to southern Europe it is also cultivated worldwide wherever the soil is well drained. In the Middle Ages it was known as Cleareye, which refers both to its ability to cleanse the eyes (the herb, not the essential oil) and its reputation for inducing visions.

It is closely related to garden sage (*Salvia officinalis*), but since it has lower levels of ketones is much safer to use. Clary Sage is known as a euphoric and is deeply relaxing for muscles and mind. It lifts you above daily cares, but at the same time is grounding, earthy and inspiring. It is said to have a progesterone like effect and can be used to regulate hormonal cycles and relieve the discomfort of heats or season.

It also helps to release energy in the lower chakras and encourages sexual activity. Last but not least, Clary Sage releases constriction in the lungs, deepening breathing and relieving fearful tension.

Principal Uses

Physical
- Alopecia
- Asthma
- Circulatory problems
- Claustrophobia
- Hormonal problems
- Tight or strained muscles

Behavioral
- Anxiety
- Changeable moods
- Claustrophobia

- Depression
- Fear

I most often use Clary Sage for:
- Restless, moody dogs, especially if there is any constriction of lungs or muscles, or claustrophobia.
- Bad tempered females, especially if they are defensive of their personal space, or become moody or uncomfortable around their hormonal cycle.

Extraction and Characteristics: Steam distilled from the flowering tops and leaves.

Fragrance: Warm, musky, sweet, green and camphoraceous.

Actions: Antifungal, antiseptic, antispasmodic, antisudorific, detoxicant, decongestant, hormone balancer (progesterone-like), neurotonic, phlebotonic, regenerative.

Safety & Cautions: Non–toxic, non-irritant, non-sensitizing. Do not mix with alcohol.

Maximum dilution 3 drops in 5 ml / 1 tsp.

Frankincense
(Boswellia Carterii)

History and Character:
Frankincense is a small tree or shrub with masses of pinnate leaves and white or pale pink flowers. It grows wild throughout the deserts of Northeast Africa. It has been an important incense in all the religions of the world since the ancient Egyptians. Frankincense slows and deepens breathing, which is why it is useful for asthma.

It is also said to "distance the mind from worries and fears". Frankincense eases the passage through major transitions, including death, and can be offered to dogs approaching the end. Frankincense also helps to let go of the past and old attachments that have outgrown their usefulness. It calms and centers the mind, allowing us to focus on the present.

Principal Uses
Physical
- Asthma
- Claustrophobia
- Diarrhea, especially if triggered by nerves
- Dry, sensitive skin
- Scars, ulcers and wounds
- Skin growths
- To ease the passage into death

Behavioral
- Anxiety and restlessness
- Noise sensitivity
- Specific fears, e.g., fireworks
- Stereotypical behavior (cribbing, pacing, spinning)

I most often use Frankincense for:

- Anxious or fearful dogs, especially if there are signs of claustrophobia (such as pacing or refusing to go into enclosed areas), asthma, or loose stools.

- Fear of fireworks and other known triggers.

- When considering euthanasia.

Extraction and Characteristics: Steam distilled from the oleo gum resin. It is a pale yellowish to green liquid.

Fragrance: Sweet, balsamic top-note and resinous, smoky bottom-note.

Actions: Analgesic, anticatarrhal, anti-depressive, anti-inflammatory, antiseptic, antioxidant, cicatrizant, energizing, expectorant, immunostimulant.

Safety & Cautions: Generally held to be non-toxic, non-irritant and non-sensitizing.

Maximum dilution 5 drops in 5 ml/1 tsp.

Fennel, Sweet
(Foeniculum Vulgare Var. Dulce)

History and Character

Fennel is a hardy perennial or biennial herb with soft, green, ferny leaves and umbrels of yellow flowers. Native to the shores of the Mediterranean it is now widely cultivated. Aromatherapy uses Sweet or garden fennel, not bitter or common fennel, which has a high level of the potentially harmful ketone, fenchone.

Traditionally, fennel has been used as a culinary herb worldwide. The Ancient Greeks used it as a diuretic to help lose weight and to promote strength. In Europe, fennel was hung over cottage doors as protection against witchcraft. It was known as an antidote for all sorts of poisons.

Strangely enough, however, snakes were said to rub against it to improve their eyesight. Perhaps due to its anti-toxic properties, fennel was said to provide courage, strength and longevity.

It is a warm, dry oil that has great affinity with the female reproductive system and the energy of nurture and care. Since it is helpful in finding ways of expressing a caring nature constructively, it is good for those who think too much, worry about the welfare of others, or have an obsessive need to nurture (sometimes manifesting as phantom pregnancy). It also helps release gas and bloating in the digestive system, and generally relieves dampness, which can lead to fatty lumps and edema.

Principal Uses

Physical
- Arthritis, rheumatism
- Constipation
- Fatty lumps
- Fluid retention
- Intestinal gas
- Phantom pregnancy

- Poisonous bites
- Problems with lactation
- Spasmodic colic
- To regulate hormonal cycles
- Urinary infections

Behavioral
- Anxiety related obsessive behavior
- Over—or under—active nurture impulses
- Those who worry about others or seek constant reassurance

I most often use Sweet Fennel for:

- Emotionally insecure animals who are over concerned with others, especially if there is a history of digestive upsets, flatulence, hormonal imbalance or fluid retention.
- Obsessive anxiety.
- Tumors and soft lumps, especially mammary.

Extraction and Characteristics: Steam distilled from the crushed seeds. The oil is a colorless to pale yellow liquid.

Fragrance: A sweet anise like fragrance, sharp green with a warm earthy undertone.

Actions: Analgesic, antibacterial, antifungal, anti-inflammatory, antiseptic, antispasmodic, cardiotonic, carminative, cholagogic, circulatory stimulant, decongestant, digestive, diuretic, emmenagogic, hormone-like, lactogenic, laxative, litholytic, estrogen like, respiratory tonic (rapid breathing).

Safety: Generally considered to be non-sensitizing, but moderately irritating to the skin. Use only in high dilutions. Do not use during pregnancy.

Maximum dilution: 1 drop in 5ml/1tsp.

Geranium
(Pelargonium Graveolens)

History and Character

A sprawling, aromatic perennial shrub with hairy serrated leaves and small pink flowers. Pelargonium graveolens is native to South Africa but widely cultivated. Until recently, the essential oil was mostly produced in Réunion (Bourbon), Egypt, Madagascar and China, with the Bourbon oil being the most prized. South Africa now produces a very good quality oil as well.

Since there is so much confusion between pelargonium, which we call geranium, and true geranium, which we call cranesbill or herb Robert, it is not clear what the historical uses of the plant were. Nevertheless, the strongest physical and energetic action of geranium oil is "to regulate". This is due to its powerful effect on the adrenal cortex, which regulates hormones and other endocrine functions.

It is one of the most Yin of the essential oils and helps us to reconnect with the feminine principle, increasing sensitivity, spontaneity, and the ability to receive. And making us feel secure in ourselves. Geranium can be used anywhere there is a lack of Yin, which is characterized by dryness, rigidity, or overheating, and is especially good for mature females.

Principal Uses

Physical

- All endocrine imbalances
- Dry or greasy flaky skin
- Facial neuralgia
- Fungal infections of the skin
- Hormone problems
- Lice and mosquitoes
- Skin problems, especially greasy dandruff

Behavioral
- Insecure, moody types
- New home or other disruptions to lifestyle

I most often use Geranium for:
- Insecure or depressed dogs who lack self confidence, especially if their moods are cyclical or their skin is over dry, greasy or unbalanced.
- Older females/adolescent males who show a lack of receptivity.

Extraction and Characteristics: Steam distilled from the leaves, stalks and flowers. The oil is a wonderful clear green color.

Fragrance: A very sweet and fresh, slightly spicy top-note, with green mid-notes and a musty, river-bottom, bottom-note.

Actions: Analgesic, antibacterial, antidiabetic, antifungal, anti-inflammatory, antiseptic, antispasmodic, astringent, cicatrizant, decongestant, digestive, hemostatic, insect repellent, phlebotonic (lymph) relaxant, tonic to liver and kidneys.

Safety & Cautions: Generally held to be non-toxic, non-irritant and non-sensitizing. It has been known to trigger dermatitis in some individuals, especially with the Bourbon type.

Maximum dilution 7 drops in 5 ml/1 tsp.

Ginger
(Zingiber Officinale)

History and Character

An erect, reed like perennial herb growing from a spreading tuberous pungent rhizome. Native to southern Asia but widely cultivated throughout the tropics. Ginger is a well known cooking spice and healing remedy that has been used for thousands of years. Best known as a digestive, it is also used for nausea and travel sickness.

Ginger is useful for overproduction of mucous, or diarrhea. Due to its deeply warming nature, ginger is often appreciated by older dogs and those who suffer from arthritis. Energetically, ginger is hot and stimulant and a restorative of Yang energy, giving a boost to those who lack physical energy. Ginger ignites those who lack confidence and the determination to carry things through, increases feelings of self worth, and lifts the despondent.

Principal Uses

Physical

- Arthritis
- Backache
- Congested lungs and sinus (white or clear mucous)
- Diarrhea
- Flatulence
- Lack of sexual performance
- Muscular aches and pains
- Pancreatic problems
- Sluggish digestion
- Soft lumps on skin
- Travel sickness

Behavioral
- Depression
- Lack of confidence

I most often use Ginger for:
- Depressed, run down dogs, especially if they have non-specific skin nodules or other symptoms of excess damp, such as diarrhea or clear mucous.
- Old dogs that feel the cold and may be stiff.

Extraction and Characteristics: Steam distilled from the unpeeled, dried root. The oil is pale yellow to amber liquid.

Fragrance: Warm, spicy, slightly earthy, pungent.

Actions: Analgesic, anticatarrhal, carminative, digestive, expectorant, general tonic, sexual tonic, stomachic.

Safety & Cautions: Generally held to be non-toxic, non-irritant, but long term use can cause sensitization. Dilute well

Maximum dilution 2 drops in 5 ml/1 tsp.

Helichrysum
(Helichrysum Italicum)

History and Character
A strongly aromatic shrub, about 60 cm./2 ft. tall with a multi branched stem of silvery, lanceolate leaves, helichrysum is native to the Mediterranean region (especially the eastern part). The small, bright yellow, daisy like flowers dry out as the plant matures, but still retain their color and fragrance. Hence the common name of everlast or *immortelle*.

Traditionally used in a decoction for migraine, chronic respiratory problems, liver ailments and all types of skin conditions, this is the best essential oil for bruises. You can practically watch the bruise fade before your eyes after applying a few drops of undiluted helichrysum. What's more, unlike the other famous bruise remedy, arnica, it can be used on broken skin to disinfect cuts.

Helichrysum has a similar effect on bruised emotions, dissolving resentment held over from past injuries. Energetically, helichrysum releases blocked energy, especially anger that has been repressed and become resentful.

Principal Uses
Physical
- Aches, pains, strains
- Allergies
- Asthma, bronchitis, chronic coughs
- Bacterial infections
- Bruises and wounds
- Burns, boils, eczema
- Hepatic congestion
- Nervous exhaustion

Behavioral
- Deeply hurt emotions
- Habitually negative behavior

- Past abuse
- Resentful, simmering anger

I most often use Helichrysum for:

- Dogs holding resentment over past ill treatment and are currently stuck in negative patterns that are counter productive. This is especially so if they have irritated skin.
- Any bumps/bruises, impact injury, rash, or burn.

Extraction and Characteristics: Steam distilled from the fresh flowers. It is a pale yellow, red tinged oil with a powerful honey like scent and a slightly bitter/pungent undertone.

Actions: Anti-allergenic, anticatarrhal, anticoagulant, antidiabetic, antifungal, antihaematomic, anti-inflammatory, antiseptic, antispasmodic, antiviral, digestive, cholagogic, cicatrizant, hepatic, mucolytic, neurotonic, phlebotonic, stimulant.

Safety & Cautions: Generally held to be non-toxic, non-irritant and non-sensitizing.

Maximum dilution 3 drops in 5 ml/1 tsp. Can be used undiluted in emergency first aid.

Juniper berry
(Juniperus Communis)

History and Character

A shrubby, evergreen tree with bluish green needles, small flowers and green or black berries, juniper is found throughout the northern hemisphere. There are several species of juniper from which an oil is produced, and their actions are different. So pay attention to the full Latin name.

Traditionally, juniper berry has been used for urinary infections, respiratory problems and gastrointestinal conditions. It also flushes out the liver and breaks down uric acid. Juniper's sharp pungent fragrance dispels negativity and since ancient times has been used for spiritual purification.

It is especially powerful with clearing out and protecting our psychic space. Juniper berry benefits those who are overwhelmed by crowds, or lack confidence in social groups, and helps to settle those who feel restless after being at "an occasion" such as a social gathering or show.

Principal Uses

Physical

- After medical procedures to cleanse the liver
- Arthritis
- Kidney infections
- Muscle cramps
- Edema
- Overworked soft tissue

Behavioral

- Nervous snappishness
- Restlessness
- Suspicion
- Those who are restless in or overwhelmed by crowds

I most often use Juniper berry for:

- Dogs who have withdrawn into themselves, often being grumpy and actively protective of their space. Especially if there is any stiffness of joints or muscles, weakening of the bladder, or a history of medical procedures requiring anesthetic.

- Those who fall apart in crowds.

Extraction and Characteristics: Steam distilled from the fresh berries. Sometimes fermented berries are used, but this is an inferior product. There is also an inferior oil made from the twigs and wood. The oil is a clear or slightly yellow mobile liquid.

Fragrance: Camphoraceous, fresh, piney, with a warm, woody undertone.

Actions: Analgesic, anti-diabetic, antiseptic, detoxicant, digestive tonic, diuretic, hypo-uremic (breaks down uric acid), litholytic, soporific.

Safety: Generally held to be non-toxic, non-irritant and non-sensitizing. It should be used with caution in patients with kidney inflammation as high levels of the diuretics 4-terpineol and terpinen-4-ol may cause irritation. Do not use in pregnancy.

Maximum dilution 3 drops in 5 ml/1 tsp.

Lavender
(Lavandula Angustifolia/Officinalis)

History and Character

An evergreen perennial herb with pale spiky leaves and violet blue flowers that rise above the main bush on slender stalks. Native to the Mediterranean but now cultivated all over the world, the best oil traditionally comes from Provence (France).

Lavender has been with us as a folk remedy for a very long time and is intimately interwoven with the development of aromatherapy as it is known today. Lavender is said to have a highly synergistic nature, strengthening the actions of other oils it is blended with. Energetically, lavender is cool and dry, soothing our brows in times of feverish emotions. It stills the heart and helps oversensitive individuals express themselves freely. It is particularly useful for those whose emotions overwhelm reason, paralyzing action or inducing hysteria.

Many countries now produce good quality lavender, and it is worth having a selection as each lavender carries the energy of the land and culture producing it. For example, lavender from England is genteel, moist and very soothing. Lavender from Israel is hot, dry and very fast acting. Lavender grown at high altitude is the most energetically refined. I call lavender Florence Nightingale, after the famous British nurse, because you can always call on it for a little light nursing or when in need of extra TLC (tender loving care), either physically or emotionally. I have also heard it referred to as the "Swiss army knife" of essential oils.

Principal Uses

Physical

- Burns
- Flea repellent
- Proud flesh
- Scars
- Sinusitis

- Stress related skin conditions
- Swellings
- To support other oils
- Wounds

Behavioral

- Nervous hysteria
- Shock
- Shyness

I most often use Lavender for:

- All types of skin conditions, especially burns and proud flesh, especially if dogs show nervous restlessness and/or have a strong need for connection.
- Shy, timid dogs who want to connect but don't dare.

Extraction and Characteristics: Steam distilled from the fresh flowering tops.

Fragrance: Sweet, herbaceous, floral, slightly camphoraceous.

Actions: Analgesic, antibacterial, antifungal, anti-inflammatory, antiseptic, antispasmodic, calmative, cardiotonic, carminative, cicatrizant, emmenagogic, hypotensive, sedative, tonic.

Safety & Cautions: Generally held to be non-toxic, non-irritant and non-sensitizing. May be applied to the skin without dilution. However, lavender oil is often adulterated.

Maximum dilution 5 drops in 5 ml/1 tsp. Can be used undiluted in emergency first aid

Lemon
(Citrus Limon)

History and Character

A small citrus tree with glossy, evergreen leaves, small white flowers, and an abundance of yellow fruit. Native to Asia, it now grows wild in the southern Mediterranean and is widely cultivated. It is a very nutritious fruit and a great pick me up.

Traditionally, it has been used to protect against typhoid, malaria and scurvy. Physically, one of lemon's strongest actions is as an immune stimulant. It also has the ability to break down excessive buildup of calcium - for example, kidney stones.

Energetically, lemon is light, cleansing, refreshing, uplifting. It sharpens focus and reduces confusion, helping to assimilate change and increase trust in one's self and others. Lemon is a simple soul with a wide range of uses and one of my personal favorites.

Principal Uses

Physical

- Bony growths
- Immune tonic
- Kidney and liver congestion
- Kidney stones
- Behavioral
- Hyper alert dogs
- Issues of trust
- Over reactive dogs

I most often use Lemon for:

- Hyperactive dogs who tend to run when scared, especially if they are underweight or prone to illness or lack trust in themselves or their owner.

- Bony growths.

Extraction and Characteristics: cold-pressed from the outer part of the fresh peel.

Fragrance: Sharp, sweet, clean with a bitter bottom note.

Actions: Anti-anemic, antibacterial, anticoagulant, antifungal, anti-inflammatory, antisclerotic, antiseptic (air), antispasmodic (stomach), antiviral, astringent, calmative, carminative, digestive, diuretic, expectorant, immunostimulant, litholytic, pancreatic stimulant, phlebotonic, stomachic.

Safety & Cautions: Non-toxic, may cause dermal irritation in some individuals. Possibly photo-toxic. Dilute below 2% on exposed skin.

Maximum dilution 3 drops in 5 ml/1 tsp.

Lemongrass
(Cymbopogon Citratus)

History and Character
Lemongrass is a fast growing tropical grass, with long sharp leaves and a thick network of roots. It has an invigorating, sharp, lemony scent, with a grassy, rooty undertone. Due to its fragrance and antiseptic properties lemongrass is commonly used in soaps and cleaning products.

In India it is also widely used in Ayurvedic medicine to: help bring down fevers; treat infectious illnesses; as a tea to calm stomach cramps; and as a pesticide and preservative for palm leaf manuscripts. Lemongrass has also traditionally been used for arthritis and muscular pain.

In 2006 researchers at Israel's University of Ben Gurion found that lemongrass caused apoptosis (programmed cell death) in cancer cells in vitro. This oil is both stimulant and sedative, clearing the mind, grounding the body and relieving anxiety.

Principal uses
Physical

- Diarrhea
- Digestive upset
- Flea and mosquito repellent
- Fungal infection
- Lymphatic drainage
- Nervous exhaustion
- Neuralgia
- Rheumatism
- Soft tissue damage
- Tumors
- Viral infections

Behavioral

- Anxiety
- Confusion
- Depression

I most often use Lemongrass for:

- In flea or fly spray, especially for dogs who tend to be stiff.
- Chronic problems of the digestive or musculo-skeletal system, especially if accompanied by depression or anxiety.

Extraction and characteristics: Steam distilled from the fresh or partially dried grass. Pale yellow, to amber liquid.

Fragrance: Fresh, sharp, lemony, with earthy undertones.

Actions: Analgesic, antidepressant, antimicrobial, antiseptic, antispasmodic, astringent, fungicidal, insecticidal, nervine, sedative (nervous system).

Safety & Cautions: While generally held to be non-toxic, there are possibilities of adverse reactions on skin. Thus use at low dilutions.

Maximum dilution 3 drops in 5 ml/1 tsp.

Manuka
(Leptospermum Scoparium)

History and Character

A medium sized shrub with small spiky leaves and pink flowers, manuka grows wild throughout New Zealand. The Maoris used various parts of it for a wide range of complaints: from head colds to fractures, burns to dysentery.

Captain Cook named it tea tree and wrote: "the leaves were used by many of us as a tea that has a very agreeable bitter taste and flavor when they are fresh, but loses some of both when they are dried". These days the plant is best known in manuka honey, which is recommended by medical practitioners for its immune stimulant and bactericidal properties, especially for topical use on wounds and burns.

The bactericidal properties of manuka are much higher in oil produced from the East Cape, New Zealand chemotype. Energetically, manuka is cleansing and nourishing and settles anxiety. These properties are very similar to tea tree oil, but manuka is softer and more feminine.

Principal Uses

Physical

- Bacterial infections and healing of wounds
- Coughs, cold and flu
- Muscular aches and pain
- Ringworm and other fungal infections
- Skin eruptions
- Ulcers and wounds, cuts and abrasions

I most often use Manuka for:

- Dogs who are run down, especially if they have eruptive skin conditions or fungal infections or tend to be anxious.
- Staphylococcus or other bacterial infections.

Extraction and Characteristics: Steam distilled from the leaves and terminal branchlets of the East Cape chemotype of Leptospermum Scoparium. It is a pale amber liquid with a slightly oily texture.

Fragrance: Pungent, herbaceous aroma with a subtle spicy undertone.

Actions: Anti-allergenic, antibacterial (especially gram+ bacteria), antifungal, antihistamine, anti- inflammatory, antiseptic, insecticidal.

Safety: Generally held to be non-toxic, non-irritant, and non-sensitizing.

Maximum dilution 5 drops in 5 ml/1 tsp. Can be used undiluted in emergency first aid.

Myrrh
(Commiphora Myrrha)

History and Character

Myrrh is a shrub or small tree with sturdy knotted branches, trifoliate aromatic leaves and small white flowers. The trunk exudes an oleoresin, which hardens into red brown tears. The trees are native to Northeast Africa and Southwest Asia, especially the desert regions of the Red Sea. The name is derived from the Arabic for 'bitter'.

Myrrh is the grand old man of essential oils, one of the first substances to be valued for its scent. The ancient Egyptians valued it as a healing unguent, and burnt it to honor the dead. The ancient Hebrews drank it with wine to prepare themselves for religious ceremonies. Jesus was offered wine laced with myrrh on the cross to diminish his suffering.

Myrrh is like a desert wind, drying out dampness and invigorating those who are slow, lethargic or run down. Myrrh frees thoughts that are caught in a pattern of restlessness, brings peace of mind, helps close wounds physically and emotionally, and creates a quiet place inside to recover from loss or rejection.

Principal Uses

Physical

- Excess mucous
- Fungal skin infections
- Gum infections (hydrosol only)
- Rain scald and mud fever
- Weeping wounds

Behavioral

- Grief, loss
- Exaggerated concern for others
- Quiet anxiety
- Sadness

- Weighed down by responsibility

I most often use Myrrh for:
- Restless dogs that worry about others, especially if they are prone to damp, oozing skin conditions or excess mucous.
- Those who are stoic about pain and past suffering, especially if they have breathing problems.

Extraction and Characteristics: Steam distilled from the crude resin or (more commonly) solvent extraction from the crude myrrh to make a resinoid. The resinoid is a thick brown viscous mass not pourable at room temperature. The essential oil is a pale amber, oily liquid that is very sticky.

Fragrance: Sweet/sharp balsamic smell, resinous and slightly camphoraceous.

Action: Antifungal, anti-inflammatory, antiseptic, antispasmodic, astringent, cardiac tonic, carminative, cicatrizant, expectorant, immunostimulant, sedative, stomachic, tonic, vulnerary.

Safety & Cautions: Non-irritant, non-sensitizing, possibly toxic in high concentrations. Avoid in pregnancy.

Maximum dilution 3 drops in 5 ml/1 tsp

Orange, sweet
(Citrus Sinensis)

History and Character

Smaller than the bitter orange that produces neroli oil, the sweet orange tree is not so hardy and has softer, broader leaves. Native to China, it is now cultivated wherever there is a Mediterranean climate. The oil is pressed out of the orange skin and is mainly produced in Israel, Brazil and North America.

The dried orange peel has been used in Chinese medicine for centuries, the sweet orange being thought to increase bronchial excretion. The tree is also a traditional sign of good luck and prosperity. In Europe the oil has been used for nervous disorders, heart problems, colic, asthma and melancholy.

Energetically, this oil is very happy, positive, young and playful. Since it is a gentle option for stomach upsets and nervousness that are not deep rooted I use it a lot with youngsters. Orange encourages a more playful outlook on life, helping to move built up stress and frustration. It is a good oil for the perfectionist and those who try too hard. It encourages a more easy going attitude.

Principal Uses

Physical

- Constipation
- Mouth ulcers
- Obesity
- Youngsters' tummy aches

Behavioral

- Anxious to please
- Depression
- Insecure
- Nervous tension
-

I most often use Sweet Orange for:

- Young dogs with a nervous disposition who feel stressed by learning to the point of explosion, especially if there is a history of stomach upsets or overeating.
- A good "helper" oil when a little lift is needed.

Extraction and Characteristics: cold-pressed out of the ripe outer peel. The oil is a pale, burnt orange, mobile liquid.

Fragrance: A sweet, fresh fruity, warm odor.

Actions: Antispasmodic, calmative, carminative, cholagogic, digestive, hepatic, stomachic.

Safety & Cautions: Generally held to be non-toxic, non-irritant and non-sensitizing. Since regular cultivation uses high levels of pesticide and can contaminate the oil it is important to use organic orange.

Maximum dilution 5 drops in 5 ml/1 tsp.

Plai
(Zingiber cassumunar)

History and Character

Approximately 60 cm/2 ft. tall, plai has grass like lancelet leaves that die annually. The flower stalk bearing white or yellow flowers grows directly from the root. The tuberous root is thick and white inside with a wonderfully characteristic ginger scent.

Plai is native to Thailand, where for centuries it has been used for medicinal purposes, particularly to combat joint and muscle pain. While closely related to "normal" ginger, it is not hot. Plai has a unique cooling action on inflamed areas, whether they are joints and muscles or kidneys and lungs.

There is some research suggesting that undiluted plai works as well as ibuprofen for pain relief in humans. Plai has also been used to counter irritable bowel syndrome and for asthma. Plai from central Thailand has a significant percentage of dimethoxyphenyl butadiene, known for its analgesic effects. Plai is energetically cooling, allowing dogs who are wound up or hot tempered to feel more grounded and trusting.

Principal uses

Physical

- Asthma
- Catarrh
- Digestive upset
- Fevers
- Inflammation of joints and muscles
- Influenza
- Respiratory problems
- Soft tissue damage, sprains and strains

Behavioral

- Agitated

- Bad tempered

- Confused

- Impatient

I most often use plai for:

- For any musculo-skeletal pain or injury, especially if dogs are bad tempered or worn down by injuries, have an occasional dry cough, or digestion is disturbed.

Extraction and characteristics: Steam distilled from the fresh or dried root.

Fragrance: Cool, green, pungent, with a hint of earth.

Actions: Analgesic, anti-neuralgic, anti-inflammatory, antiseptic, antispasmodic, antitoxic, antiviral, carminative, digestive, diuretic, febrifuge, laxative, rubefacient, stimulant, tonic and vermifuge.

Safety & Cautions: No known safety issues.

Maximum dilution 5 drops in 5 ml/1 tsp.

Rosalina
(Melaleuca Ericifolia)

History and Character

Native to Australia, Rosalina is a huge shrub, 6-9 m/20-30 ft. tall,with a bushy top and grayish papery bark, with soft, alternate, smooth and narrow linear leaves. Similar to Melaleuca alternifolia, rosalina readily produces new top growth after severe cutting. It grows in low lying swamps, along creeks and behind sand dunes. It does all the same things as tea tree (melaleuca alternifolia), but its high linalol content makes it easy on the skin. It is a gentle Yin oil, very cooling and relaxing and tender. Thus I very much prefer it for dogs.

Principal Uses

Physical

- Bladder infections

- Boils

- Fevers

- Respiratory infections

- Wounds

I most often use Rosalina for:

- Infected wounds or respiratory conditions, especially if the immune system is low due to stress.

Extraction and Characteristics: Steam distilled from leaves and small twigs.

Fragrance: Sharp, camphoraceous, slightly sweet herbaceous.

Actions: Antibacterial, anti-inflammatory, antiseptic, detoxicant, expectorant, febrifuge, sedative.

Safety & Cautions: Generally held to be non-toxic, non-irritant and non-sensitizing.

Maximum dilution 3 drops in 5 ml/1 tsp. Can be used undiluted in emergency first aid.

Rosemary
(Rosmarinus Officinalis)

History and Character
A strongly aromatic evergreen shrub up to 2 m/6 ft. tall, Rosemary is native to the Mediterranean. But it is widely cultivated as a culinary herb. It has an affinity to the head, stimulating the brain and encouraging hair growth. The old saying "Rosemary for remembrance" derives from its ability to enhance concentration and brain activity. But also because it was burnt at the funerals of Greeks and Romans.

In the Middle Ages in France, rosemary was burnt to disinfect the air in hospitals. Since it was reputed to strengthen body and brain, it was also used as a general panacea. Energetically, rosemary is a very stimulating herb, but also strongly earthed and with a "can do" attitude. It boosts confidence and courage in those suffering from extreme self doubt .

Principal Uses
Physical
- Hair loss or patchy coats
- Joint disease
- Muscular pain
- Respiratory congestion
- Sluggish circulation

Behavioral
- Disconnected emotionally or mentally
- Lack of confidence
- Nervous dogs

I most often use Rosemary for:
- Nervous dogs with patchy coats, who lack confidence in their abilities (often manifesting as an inability to concentrate).

Extraction and Characteristics: Steam distilled from the fresh flowering tops and leaves. The oil is a colorless to pale yellow liquid.

Fragrance: Green-herbaceous, camphoraceous, slightly sweet and warm.

Actions: Analgesic, antibacterial, antifungal, anti-inflammatory, antiseptic, antispasmodic, antitussive, antiviral, cardiotonic, carminative, choleretic, cicatrizant, detoxicant, digestive, diuretic, emmenagogic, enuresis, hyperglycemic, hypertensor, hypotensive, litholytic, lowers cholesterol, mucolytic, neuromuscular, neurotonic, sexual tonic, stimulant (adrenal cortex), venous decongestant.

Safety & Cautions: Generally held to be non-toxic, non-irritant and non-sensitizing. Use in high concentrations. There are conflicting opinions as to its safety in pregnancy and epilepsy, I recommend not to using it in either.

Maximum dilution 2 drops in 5 ml/1 tsp.

Spearmint
(Mentha Spicata)

History and Character

A creeping perennial herb with bright green leaves and spires of white or pale pink flowers, Spearmint is native to Europe. But it is also widely cultivated and valued as a food flavoring. Similar to peppermint in its ability to stimulate digestion and circulation, ease breathing and clear the mind. But it is gentler, more nurturing and less penetrating, softer, thus making it very suitable for use with youngsters and oldsters. It soothes away problems rather than cutting through them and is excellent for dull insistent pain of any sort.

Principal Uses

Physical
- Allergy related respiratory problems
- Anesthetic
- Circulatory problems, muscle spasms and cramps
- Digestive disorders
- Flatulence and nausea
- Clearing respiratory mucous
- Young dogs

Behavior
- Hotheads
- Impulsive Behavior
- Lack of focus

I most often use Spearmint for:
- Young dogs with digestive or respiratory problems, especially if they are impulsive.
- Older dogs with persistent dull pain internally or externally.

Extraction and Characteristics: Steam distilled from the flowering tops. The oil is a pale yellow to green liquid.

Fragrance: Warm, sweet herbaceous, spicy green fragrance.

Actions: Anesthetic (local), antiseptic, antispasmodic, astringent, carminative, decongestant, digestive, diuretic, expectorant, febrifuge, hepatic, neurotonic, stimulant, stomachic, tonic.

Safety & Cautions: Generally held to be non-toxic, non-irritant and non-sensitizing.

Maximum dilution 5 drops in 5 ml/1 tsp.

Vetiver
(Vetiveria Zizanoides)

History and Character:
A tall tropical grass with scented tufts and a spreading root system, Vetiver is native to Southern India (where it is known as the Oil of Tranquility), Indonesia and Sri Lanka. It is, however, currently mostly cultivated in Java, Haiti and Réunion. Traditionally, Indians have used vetiver as a vermin repellent and woven into aromatic matting for their houses.

The Indians anoint themselves with the oil in the hot season to help keep them cool, and in Ayurvedic medicine it is used for joint problems and eczema. Energetically, vetiver is the "Earth mother" oil, nurturing, calming and reassuring. It helps us gather together scattered energies and get grounded and brings us back to the present.

I call it the "Labrador oil" as I commonly use it for the over enthusiastic love me, love me behavior that is typical of Labrador retrievers. Conversely, it is also useful for underweight dogs who are apologetic about their existence.

Principal Uses
Physical
- Anemia
- Physically run down
- Underweight for no good reason

Behavioral
- Emotional insecurity
- Perfectionists
- Pushy dogs who try to walk all over you
- Restlessness
- Ungrounded dogs who don't know where they begin and end

I most often use vetiver for:

- Dogs who walk all over you in enthusiasm or fear, or don't know where their feet are, tend to knock things over, or step on you, and seek constant reassurance.

- Dogs who are thin despite eating well and need nourishment.

Extraction and Characteristics: Steam distilled from the roots and rootlets. The oil is viscous and dark amber.

Fragrance: Smoky, wet earth, with sweet overtones.

Actions: Anti-anemic, antiseptic, circulatory tonic, emmenagogic, glandular tonic (pancreatic secretion), immunostimulant.

Safety & Cautions: Generally held to be non-toxic, non-irritant and non-sensitizing.

Maximum dilution 3 drops in 5 ml/1 tsp.

Yarrow
(Achillea Millefolium)

History and Character

Yarrow is a perennial herb growing up to 1 meter/3 ft. tall, but more usually less than half this height. It has a basal rosette of fern like leaves and a tall stem bearing a tight knit cluster of white to pale pink flowers that look like a shield. Protection is one of its signatures. Native to Eurasia and found in hedgerows throughout Britain, it has naturalized in most temperate zones. But the chamazulene content is highest in oil distilled in Eastern Europe.

Yarrow was reputed to have been used by Achilles (hence the name) for wounds caused by iron weapons. The stalks are traditionally used for reading the *I-Ching*. Yarrow helps release energy held around physical and emotional scars. In short, past traumas, especially when they manifest as a combination of anger and fear. Yarrow is one of the essential oils I use most commonly for dogs, especially the troubled kind with an unknown history. Or if, because of behavior or scars, I suspect past traumas of any kind.

Principal Uses
Physical

- Allergies

- Arthritis

- Ear infections

- Inflammations

- Scars

- Skin problems of all kinds

- Sprains and strains

- Urinary infections

- Wounds

Behavioral
- Emotional release around scars
- Fearful anger
- Past abuse

I most often use Yarrow for:
- Dogs whose past history is unknown, especially if they are showing behavioral problems, or if there is a history of physical or emotional traumas.
- First aid to stop bleeding.
- As an anti-inflammatory.

Extraction and Characteristics: Steam distilled from the dried herb. The best oil is a deep blue.

Fragrance: Sweet, herbaceous, spicy, with a soft woody dryout.

Actions: Anti-allergenic, anti-inflammatory, antiseptic, antispasmodic, carminative, expectorant, febrifuge, hemostatic, hypotensive.

Safety: Generally held to be non-toxic, non-irritant and non-sensitizing. One of the few oils you can use undiluted. Avoid in pregnancy and young children. Yarrow can occasionally trigger "acting out" of a past trauma when used for the first time.

Maximum dilution 5 drops in 5 ml/1 tsp. Can be used undiluted in emergency first aid.

Ylang-ylang
(Cananga Odorata)

History and Character
Ylang-ylang is a tall tropical tree with large shiny leaves and fragrant tender flowers, which can be pink or yellow. The yellow flowers are considered best for essential oil. Ylang-ylang is native to tropical Asia, but the major oil producers are in Madagascar, Réunion and the Comoro Islands.

In Indonesia the flowers are spread on the bed of newlyweds. It has also been used to encourage hair growth, combat fever (including malaria) and fight infections. Energetically, it is a deeply calming oil, slowing heart rate and breathing and helping in situations where emotions overwhelm reason. It boosts self confidence and is great for young dogs who are having hierarchy issues, or excessive sex drive.

Principal Uses
Physical
- Tachycardia
- Hypopnea
- Hair growth

Behavioral
- Sexual anxiety
- Stereotypical behavior
- Young dogs lacking self confidence

I most often use Ylang-ylang for:
- Young dogs who are nervous, restless, or lack confidence, especially if it is related to hierarchical problems, or when there is hair loss.

Extraction and Characteristics

Steam distilled from the freshly picked flowers. The first hour of distillation produces what is known as Ylang-ylang extra, which is of a superior quality. Ylang-ylang 1, 2 and complete are considered inferior. The oil is a pale yellowish liquid.

Fragrance: Intensely sweet floral, balsamic, spicy.

Actions: Antidepressant, antiseptic, aphrodisiac, euphoric, hypotensive, sedative and tonic.

Safety & Cautions: Generally held to be non-toxic, non-irritant and non-sensitizing.

Maximum dilution 3 drops in 5 ml/1 tsp.

HYDROSOL PROFILES

Remember, you can always replace an essential oil with its hydrosol and achieve the same therapeutic result more gently. These are hydrosols that I have not profiled as essential oils. Stability is an indication of shelf life, the higher the stability the longer the shelf life, with three years being the outside limit.

Cornflower
(Centaurea Cyanus)
History & Character
The cornflower is an annual flowering plant, native to Europe, also known as bachelor's button, bluebottle, boutonniere flower, and hurtsickle. A striking bright blue flower, that retains its color when dried, it is grown in gardens worldwide. Historically young men wore cornflowers when in love, if the flower faded it meant their love was not returned. The most common use for this herb is for eye care. It soothes irritated eye and can reduce the inflammation of conjunctivitis. It is also mildly antibacterial. It is a gently soothing herb and can be used to soothe itching and soften skin. Since there is no essential oil of cornflower this hydrosol is particularly useful.

The fragrance is fresh and intriguing, quite sharp, with a slightly lemony/green edge.

Therapeutic uses
Physical
- Bruises,
- Hair conditioner.
- Hydrating wound wash
- Irritated eyes, use as an eyewash.
- Liver tonic

Stability: Low to moderate.
Safety & Cautions: Do not use in pregnancy.

Eucalyptus
(Eucalyptus Globulus)

History and character

Eucalyptus are tall evergreen trees with grayish blue leaves that become yellow with age, and a pale trunk with strips of colored bark that flakes off. Eucalyptus trees are native to Australia but have been introduced around the world. The eucalyptus tree draws up great quantities of water, drying out swamps so they can be farmed. The trees also release vapor loaded with the antiseptic essential oil, which repels mosquitoes carrying the malarial fever often found in swampy areas. You can spray or rub the hydrosol into your dog's coat to repel mosquitoes.

Traditionally the aborigines used eucalyptus to treat infections and fevers especially as a fumigant. Eucalyptus has a penetrating and drying energy, which dispels congestion of the lungs and lifts melancholy.

Eucalyptus clears out frustrated energy and unconscious, stagnated feelings, allowing us to breathe freely physically and emotionally.

The smell of eucalyptus hydrosol is sweet, much lighter and less penetrating than the essential oil. But to my nose has a slightly sickly undertone. The taste is sharp and tingly with a distinctly green flavor. It is drying, both topically and energetically. Dogs prefer the hydrosol to the essential oil.

Principal uses

Physical

- Coughs
- Fly/mosquito repellent
- Immune stimulant
- Inhibits the spread of airborne infection
- Reduces fever
- Respiratory problems

- Sinus infection

Behavior
- Claustrophobia
- Frustration

Stability: Medium to high
Safety & Cautions: Do not apply to sensitive skin.

Lemon Balm
(Melissa Officinalis)

History and Character

This plant originated in the Mediterranean region but is now widely cultivated. It is a leafy perennial, with small white-pink flowers. It grows to about 60 cm (2 feet) and likes well drained sandy soil with a high iron content. In the right conditions the plant can be an invasive weed.

The plant yields very little essential oil, so is one of the most expensive on the market and widely adulterated. Because of this I use the hydrosol instead of the essential oil.

Melissa has an illustrious past and is often mentioned by traditional medics, it was described by John Evelyn (1620 -1706) as "sovereign for the brain, strengthening the memory, and powerfully chasing away melancholy". Melissa means honey bee in Greek, because they love the nectar of this herb.

Melissa is a strong anti-viral and immune stimulant. It is also used as a nerve sedative, digestive aid, antidepressant, and to regulate hormonal cycles. Melissa is tonic to the heart, slowing the heartbeat, and reducing blood pressure. I use it mainly for its powerful immune stimulant properties and for calming nerves, as it is very relaxing without being sedative. In humans, it has been used successfully for ADHD, reducing hyperactivity and increasing focus.

This hydrosol strengthens ones sense of self, and is particularly suited to dogs who are over-sensitive, or easily traumatized by confrontation. Lemon balm (or Melissa) hydrosol has a light, sweet, citrus green fragrance, very refreshing and uplifting with a sharp edge.

Principle uses
Physical
- Immune stimulant
- Calming nerves, relaxing without being sedative
- Digestive aid, use in moderation.

Behavioral
- Hyperactivity
- Confused
- Lack of focus
- Nervous

Stability: Moderate
Safety & Cautions: Don't use in cases of hypotension, or glaucoma.

Neroli (Orange blossom)
(Citrus Aurantium, var. Amara)

History and Character
The orange tree is a medium size flowering citrus, native to China, but now widely cultivated in any Mediterranean climate. It has glossy green, heart-shaped leaves, a smooth grey bark and masses of fragrant white flowers. Neroli is produced by steam distillation from the flowers of the tree. It is another costly essential oil that can easily be replaced with its hydrosol.

The oil is said to be named after an Italian princess who introduced the fragrance to Italian society in the 17th century. The fragrance is a classic floral note in perfumery. In the Middle East, orange blossom water is used for fainting fits and shock. Neroli has a powerful ability to reconnect body and mind after shock from emotional or physical trauma and is a 'must have' in the first aid kit.

Neroli is highly uplifting, calming and steadies the nerves, (useful before vet visits, or other situations that provoke anxiety). Neroli heals sorrow held in the heart and eases the pain of loss or separation from a loved one.

The hydrosol has an intensely floral fragrance with more of a detectable bitter edge than the oil. It is highly complex and much more easily assimilated when diluted.

Principle uses
Physical
- Gas or bloating
- Internally as a support for itchy skin caused by food intolerance
- Shock
- Steadies the heart physically and emotionally

Behavioral
- Before something stressful like traveling
- Heartbreak
- Hysterical fear

- Sadness
- Where emotion has overcome the "civilized mind".

Stability: High
Safety & Cautions: It is potentially drying to the skin Don't use in cases of hypotension.

Peppermint
(Mentha Piperita)

History and Character

A perennial herb up to 1 m/3 ft high with strong underground runners, green stems and leaves. There is also a black peppermint which has dark green serrated leaves and purplish stems. Peppermint has a long history of medicinal and culinary use. The essential oil is classified as a medicine for digestive problems, such as colitis and irritable bowel syndrome.

Energetically, peppermint is invigorating and awakening, bringing things into focus mentally and emotionally. It helps animals to be clear about their boundaries so it is easy to take in and give out without defensiveness and with discrimination.

Full of life with a wonderful fresh green, zingy fragrance, the hydrosol is softer than most peppermint essential oils. Dogs often find peppermint essential oil too strong, and prefer the hydrosol.

Principle uses

Physical
- Colitis
- Flatulence
- Heat stroke
- Indigestion
- Inflamed soft tissue
- Irritable bowel syndrome
- Nausea

Behavioral
- Defensive of personal space
- Hyperactivity
- Irritability
- Scatty

Stability: Low

Safety & Cautions: Do not use with very young.

Rose
(Rosa Damascena)
History and Character

Rose hydrosol comes from the Damask Rose, a bush rose up to 2 m/6 ft high with highly fragrant, pink, 36-petalled blooms. Originally a product of the orient, roses are now cherished all over the world, however the best oil is produced in Bulgaria and some parts of Turkey.

'The queen of flowers', dedicated to Aphrodite, rose is one of the most yin aromatics and its cooling properties are second to none. It releases energy blocked because of emotional wounds, especially when this manifests as resentfulness and an attitude of, "I will reject you before you can reject me". It promotes self-love and allows the heart to be receptive, restoring trust in oneself and others. It also has a powerful effect on the hormonal system and balances the physical and emotional body.

The hydrosol smells much like the essential oil, although slightly sweeter. This is another case where the essential oil is expensive, and the hydrosol just as effective, if not more so.

Principle uses
Physical
- Astringent and cooling for the skin
- Eye wash to soothe redness and irritation
- Hormone balancer
- Post-natal recovery

Behavioral
- Loss of trust
- Resentful anger
- Self-abuse
- Those whose hearts have closed due to poor treatment

Stability: High

Safety & Cautions: Don't use during pregnancy, except after labor has started.

Tea tree
(Melaleuca Alternifolia)

History and character

Tea tree is a low growing tree with needle-like leaves and small yellow or purplish flowers. Native to Australia, the Aboriginal people used its leaves in a tea for fevers, colds, and headaches. It has been extensively researched in recent years and found to be a powerful immunostimulant and active against bacteria, fungi and viruses. Energetically, it is tremendously cleansing, fortifying the lungs and giving confidence. It is useful for those who feel victimized or unable to cope with worldly matters.

Despite its popularity in dog shampoos and the like, Tea tree essential oil can be dangerous to dogs, causing temporary paralysis. For this reason I only use the hydrosol. It is an effective wound wash. It is also a good hydrosol to make available in water when there is a virus going around.

Principle uses

Physical
- Wound disinfectant
- Skin infections
- Boils
- Abscesses
- Immune stimulant
- Fever

Behavioral
- Confusion about boundaries
- Self protective

Stability: Medium to high
Safety & Cautions: None known

Thyme
(Thymus Vulgaris)

History and Character

Thyme is a small, evergreen shrub with tiny fragrant leaves and woody stems. Thyme is native to the hot, rocky slopes of the Mediterranean but is cultivated throughout the world. Because of its anti-bacterial nature, the Egyptians used it for embalming. The Greeks used it to clean the air of infection. It was widely used as a cooking herb, especially to preserve meat.

In Western herbal lore, thyme has been used for respiratory infections and digestive problems. The essential oil is too harsh for most dogs. The hydrosol is an effective, gentle disinfectant, internally and externally.

Energetically, thyme is very warm and dry. It inspires fearlessness and confidence in the world. I call it the Brave oil and use it to help timid dogs face their fears. It works especially well for dogs who bark and act aggressive, then run away. They feel they must be brave but are not up to the job.

Thyme hydrosol has a warm, dry, herbaceous fragrance much like the plant at the height of summer.

Principle uses:
Physical
- Antibacterial wound wash
- Bad breath
- Dermal infections, with excessive moisture
- Digestive problems
- Infected wounds

Behavioral
- Timid dogs
- Fearful barking
- Aggressive self protection

Stability: High
Safety & Cautions: May be mildly irritant to mucous membranes.

Witch hazel
(Hamamelis Virginiana)

History and Character

Hamamelis virginiana is a small deciduous tree or shrub, native to the Eastern part of North America. It flourishes on shaded north-facing slopes. It was used extensively by Native Americans as a decoction to treat inflammation, swellings and tumors. The name comes from an Old English word meaning pliable, but may also be influenced by the use of the forked twigs as divining rods.

Witch-hazel is highly astringent and the earliest works on American medicinal plants included its use to treat eye inflammations, hemorrhoids, bites, stings and skin sores, diarrhea and dysentery. I remember its smell from childhood as my mothers favorite first aid remedy, for bruises and scrapes. It is considered one of the best herbs to stem internal and external bleeding.

In vitro research shows witch hazel to have significant anti-viral activity and be anti-inflammatory. Witch hazel has also been found to be effective in vitro against periodontal bacteria. This is another hydrosol with no equivalent essential oil and but is irreplaceable in the 1st aid box.

Energetically witch hazel is clean and clarifying, with a sharp uplifting woody fragrance. It is emotionally relaxing and can soothe restless irritation. It is delicate and enlivening.

Principle uses
Physical

- Antiseptic
- Insect bites
- Broken capillaries and bruises
- Heals wounds
- Soothing for all types of skin complaints, particularly eczema.
- Ulcers

Behavioral
- Irritability
- Restlessness
- Self-pity

Stability: Unstable, lasts only 4 months or so.

Safety & Cautions: Do not use commercially available witch hazel as it always contains alcohol. Not for internal use.

HERBAL & CARRIER OIL PROFILES

Calendula *M
(Calendula Officinalis)

History and Character

Calendula, also known as marigold, is a cheerful presence in gardens across the globe. It grows easily in any soil and since it is reputed to help keep vegetables free from pests, it is used as a companion plant in the vegetable garden. The double orange flowers are the best ones to use for macerating. The oil takes on their beautiful golden color.

Calendula is a valuable healer, and as there is no distilled essential oil (there is a CO_2 extract), the macerated oil is particularly useful. I use calendula often as a carrier oil, food supplement for stomach and fungal skin problems, and for wiping out "gunky" ears.

Synonym: Marigold oil (*Tagetes glandulifera*) is also known as marigold. So check the full Latin name when purchasing.

Principle uses

External
- Bruises and capillary damage
- Dry, cracked skin
- Fungal infections
- Slow healing wounds

Internal
- Gall bladder complaints
- Hormonal problems
- Indigestion
- Ulcers

Emotional energy: Uplifting, cheerful, comforting
Stability: Medium
Safety & Cautions: No known contraindications. Do not confuse with oil from *Tagetes patula*.

Comfrey oil *M
(Symphytum officinale)

History and Character

Comfrey's large hairy leaves and delicate purplish pink flowers are a common sight throughout Europe, but especially in the British Isles. The macerated oil can be made from the roots or leaves of this sturdy plant, or both. Comfrey is a well known healer's plant, having been used extensively in herbal medicine. One of its common names is Knitbone due to its ability to speed the healing of broken bones, bruises and wounds. It was also traditionally used for irritable coughs and chronic lung conditions.

Principle uses
External

- Broken bones
- Scar tissue and proud flesh
- Strengthens the lungs
- Traumatic injury

Emotional energy: Heals past hurt, helps to move on, strengthening
Stability: Medium
Safety & Cautions: Do not use on puncture wounds or other very deep wounds. Over consumption of the root has caused cancer in mice.

Coconut Oil
Cocus Nucifera

History and Character

Coconut oil is extracted from the fruit of the coconut tree, a large, hard shelled nut, that grows in clusters at the top of the trunk. The interior of the nut is white and smooth. Coconut is a traditional food staple in tropical climates. It has also been used for skin and hair care.

More recently research has shown that the high lauric acid content of **virgin** coconut oil is anti-inflammatory, antimicrobial, antioxidant and supports immune function. The only other substance with such high levels of lauric acid is breast milk. Virgin coconut oil is solid below 24C/76F.

Fractionated coconut has had the lauric acid removed, thus it stays liquid at all temperatures, making it easier to use. It can be useful as a neutral carrier oil or a lightweight emollient. However it is a poor substitute for the whole virgin oil, which contains the true therapeutic properties of the plant plus all vitamins, anti-oxidants and minerals. Coconut oil is cooling, soothing and nourishing, a very yin oil that can be used internally and externally for yeast infections and hot skin irritation.

Principle uses (referring to the virgin oil)

External
- Burns
- Cracked skin
- Fungal infections

Internal
- Yeast infections
- Coat conditioner
- Immune support

Emotional energy: Calms nervous irritability, impulsive behavior
Stability: High
Safety & Cautions: No known contraindications.

Hemp seed oil
(Cannabis sativa)

History and Character

Hemp seed oil is extracted from the seeds of the controversial cannabis plant. While the oil does not contain the psychoactive properties of the drug, it is, nevertheless, relaxing, warming and comforting. It has a strong nutty flavor, a high gamma linoleic acid (GLA) content and is nutritionally high in protein. The same plant is used for making a strong, pliable material or rope and hemp seed oil is a great carrier oil for dogs who are having a hard time "holding it together", physically or emotionally.

Principle uses
Internal

- Anxiety
- Arthritis
- Degenerative diseases
- Dry skin
- Eczema
- General weakness

Emotional energy: Warming, gives sense of security, grounding, relaxing
Stability: Low
Safety & Cautions: None known

Hypericum (St John's Wort) *M
(Hypericum Perforatum)

History and Character

Hypericum oil is an amazing blood red color due to the presence of hypericin, an effective antiviral agent. It is made macerating the buds and flowers picked at noon in mid-summer. In times gone by this plant was thought to protect against evil spirits, something often said of plants now known to have a strong psychological effect. St John's Wort is often used as a natural substitute for Prozac. Medieval Knights used it on sword wounds. It is now scientifically proven to be antibacterial and beneficial to wounds where there is nerve damage.

Principle uses

External

- Arthritis
- Bruises
- Burns
- Inflamed nerve conditions, such as sciatica
- Skin inflammations
- Wounds

Internal

- Unpredictable moods
- Depression
- Extreme nervousness

Emotional energy: Balancing, soothing, cooling

Safety & Cautions: Ingestion of high doses of hypericum can cause photo-sensitization in light skinned dogs.

Jojoba oil (wax)
(Simmondsia Sinensis)

History and Character

The jojoba plant is native to the deserts of the southwest US. It is a small leathery plant that takes 12 years to reach maturity and can be planted to prevent arid land becoming desert. The plant does not, strictly speaking, produce oil, but wax, which is highly stable, remaining unchanged for a period of years. It has very little odor and is nourishing to the skin. But I most often use it as a neutral carrier oil for emotional problems.

Principle uses
External

- Moisturizing to the skin
- Anti-inflammatory
- Arthritis and rheumatism
- Hair conditioner

Internal

- Carrier oil for emotional problems

Emotional energy: Neutral, smooth
Stability: High
Safety & Cautions: Jojoba oil fed to rats causes changes to histological and enzymatic activity. Do not use as a food supplement. Contact dermatitis has been reported.

Neem seed oil
(Azadirachta indica)

History and Character

The neem tree is known in India as "the village pharmacy". For more than 4,500 years traditional healers have used its bark, seeds, leaves, fruit, gum and oils for dozens of internal and external medical treatments. The most common historical uses of neem were for skin diseases, inflammation, fevers and as an antiparasitic.

In India it is claimed to be contraceptive. Neem oil is effective against at least 200 insects. It is apparently so distasteful that most of them won't eat a plant treated with it. But if they do, it throws their hormones into disarray, fatally preventing them from shedding their outgrown skins.

Principle uses

External

- Arthritis
- Eczema
- Flea, tick and mosquito repellent
- Rheumatism and arthritis
- Ringworm
- Scabies

Internal

- Antiparasitic

Emotional energy: Cooling, clarifying, sharp.

Safety & Cautions: Although the hormonal effect shown on insects has not been seen to affect mammals, do not use in pregnancy.

Sunflower oil
(Helianthus anuus L)

History and Character
Sunflower oil is another of the "neutral" oils, as it is essentially odorless. Since there is so much commercial production of sunflower oil it is really important to buy organic cold-pressed oil. If I were only allowed to have one carrier oil, this would be it.

Therapeutic uses
External
- Bruises
- Rhinitis and sinusitis
- Skin ulcers

Internal
- A carrier oil for emotional problems

Emotional energy: Neutral, supportive
Safety & Cautions: None known

AROMATIC CROSS REFERENCE CHART

Essential Oil	Physical indicators	Emotional Indicators	Common Uses
Angelica root *Angelica archangelica*	Heart disturbances, sluggish digestion, loss of appetite, hepatitis, fungal infection, immune problems, shortness of breath.	Hysteria, "switched off"', nervous, fearful, hyperactive.	For dogs who reject healing, early trauma, fear, debilitation, multiple problems.
Bergamot *Citrus aurantium, subsp, bergamia*	Tumors and growths, warts, sarcoids, bacterial infection of lungs or urinary tract, hormone imbalance, viral infection.	Depression, mood swings.	Warts/tumors, infections of lungs or genito-urinary tract, balancing emotions, post parturition.
Cajeput *Melaleuca cajeputi Powell*	Bronchitis, chronic coughs, infections, strains, sprains, tight muscles.	Obsessive, compulsive.	Arthritis, lung infections, compulsive habits.
Carrot seed *Daucus carota*	Poor skin/nails, underweight, heart problems, cuts and bruises, liver damage.	Despondent, sense of abandonment.	Malnutrition, skin and coat, slow healing wounds, abandonment, hemorrhage.
Cedarwood **Atlas** *Cedrus Atlantica*	Cough with white mucous, fleas, general tonic, kidney problems, stiffness, dandruff, hair loss.	Insecure, timid, ungrounded.	Coughs, backache, edema, genito-urinary, timidity, moving home.

Essential Oil	Physical indicators	Emotional Indicators	Common Uses
Chamomile Roman *Anthemis nobilis*	Nervous stomach, irritable skin, red eyes, runny eyes.	High strung, nervous, tantrums.	Nervousness, skin problems, nervous upset stomach, angry outbursts, problems with children.
Clary Sage *Salvia sclarea*	Tight muscles, respiratory distress, shortness of breath, dry skin, hormonal imbalance.	Fearful, over reactive, tense.	Asthma, muscle spasm, hormonal imbalance, tension, claustrophobia, fear.
Fennel *Foeniculum vulgare var., dulce.*	Flatulence, fatty lumps, lack/excess of milk, indigestion, excess hormones, poisoning.	Worry, exaggerated concern about others, emotionally needy.	False pregnancy, lactation problems, stomach upset, fluid retention, lipomas, flatulence, obesity.
Frankincense *Boswellia carterii*	Shortness of breath, nervous digestive upsets, dry, flaky skin, scars, growths.	Nervous fear, specific fears.	Fireworks, diarrhea, asthma, lice, nervous cough, break with past, tumors, skin repair.
Geranium *Pelargonium graveolens*	Hormonal imbalance, dandruff, endocrine imbalance, sluggish liver/kidneys.	Mood swings, overwhelmed insecure.	Hormonal problems, insecurity, new home, flaky skin, lice.
Ginger *Zingiber officinale*	Arthritis, cold sensitive, muscle stiffness, sore back, lung congestion, digestive.	Depression, self protective, overwhelmed by life, no self-confidence.	Sluggish digestion/ circulation, travel sickness, weakness, stiff joints, old dogs, lack of willpower.
Helichrysum *Helichrysum Italicum*	Traumatic injury, allergies, run down, multiple problems, congestion, bruising, tendon injuries.	Deep emotional wounds, resentment	Bruises, damaged tissue, past trauma, allergies.

Essential Oil	Physical indicators	Emotional Indicators	Common Uses
Juniper berry *Juniperus communis*	Arthritis, muscle strain, soft tissue damage, weak kidneys, sluggish systems.	Disturbed mind, unsettled, aloof, gloomy, worried about themselves.	Arthritis, after hard work, post-op, soft tissue damage, liver congestion, clearing mind, psychic protection
Lavender *Lavandula angustifolia*	Accidents, sensitive skin, heart palpitations.	Restless anxiety, mood swings, nervousness, shyness.	Wounds, burns, proud flesh, hot spots, skin damage, scars, hysteria, nervousness
Lemon *Citrus limon*	Run down, sluggish liver and kidneys, arthritis, ringbone, immune problems.	Slight depression, lack of trust in self or others, confusion, lack of focus.	Kidney stones, bony growths, immune disease, run down, kidney disease, lack of trust, multiple homes.
Lemon *Citrus limon*	Run down, sluggish liver and kidneys, arthritis, ringbone, immune problems.	Slight depression, lack of trust in self or others, confusion, lack of focus.	Kidney stones, bony growths, immune disease, run down, kidney disease, lack of trust, multiple homes.
Lemongrass *Cymbopogon citratus*	Compromised immune system, growths, muscle pain, arthritis.	Emotionally needy, unfocused, insecure, worried.	Fly/flea repellent, tumors, depression, confusion, pain.
Manuka *Leptospermum scoparium*	Skin problems, allergies, wounds, nervous respiratory disorders and lung infections.	Withdrawn, self protective.	Bacterial infection, skin problems, colds and flu, wounds and cuts.
Myrrh *Commiphora myrrha*	Oozing skin conditions, chronic coughs, diarrhea.	Overwhelmed with care, aloof, restless.	Fungal infections, weeping skin, persistent wet cough, mud-fever, hotspots.

Essential Oil	Physical indicators	Emotional Indicators	Common Uses
Orange, sweet *Citrus sinensis*	Indigestion, juvenile colic, mouth ulcers, gas.	Nervousness, depression.	Nervous tension especially in youngsters, obesity.
Plai *Zingiber cassumunar*	Chronic pain, acute pain, tendon damage, nerve damage, digestive cramps.	Hot headed, fearful anger, apathetic, stubborn.	Pain, soft tissue damage, asthma, boney growths, irritable bowel.
Rosalina *Melaleuca ericifolia*	Skin and lung infections, convulsions.	Fretful, protective	Wounds, skin disorders, coughs and colds, yeast infection, infections.
Rosemary *Rosmarinus officinalis*	Muscle pain, general sluggishness, clumsiness, hair loss	Hard to connect with, self critical, no sense of self.	Alopecia, convalescence, muscle strain, sinus/lung congestion, lack of concentration,
Spearmint *Mentha spicata*	Pain, digestive upsets, chronic pain, chronic dry cough.	Hyper sensitive, troubled by life, impulsive.	Digestive disorders with flatulence, respiratory mucous, muscle spasms.
Vetiver *Vetiveria zizanoides*	Under/over-weight, general stiffness and discomfort, anemia.	Flighty, hyper excitable, clumsy, knocks into you.	Hyper excitability, pushy, "no sense of their feet", weak constitution, debility.
Yarrow *Achillea millefolium*	Injuries of all types, self harm, allergies, irritated skin, liver or kidney congestion.	Past trauma, fearful anger, past abuse, unknown life story.	Emotional/physical trauma, wounds, inflammation, itchy skin, allergies, insect bites.
Ylang-ylang *Cananga odorata*	High blood pressure, loss of libido, sensitive skin, hair loss.	Nervous, insecure, no self confidence, no *joie de vivre*.	Young dogs with hierarchy issues, dry skin, nervousness, hypernea.

AROMATICS FOR SPECIFIC CONDITIONS

Condition	Essential oil/ hydrosol	Carrier oil
Musculo-skeletal problems, circulation, muscles, joints		
Aches and Pains	Cajeput, carrot seed, cedarwood, clary sage, chamomile, ginger, helichrysum, spearmint, plai, yarrow	Calendula, comfrey, hemp, hypericum,
Arthritis	Angelica Root, cajeput, carrot seed, cedarwood, fennel, ginger, juniper berry, plai, yarrow	Comfrey, hemp, hypericum, neem
Bony Growths	Helichrysum, lemon, plai	Comfrey
Bruising	Chamomile, helichrysum, lavender, witch hazel	Comfrey, calendula, sunflower
Bursitis	Angelica root, cedarwood, helichrysum, juniper berry, yarrow	Comfrey, sunflower, calendula, neem
Broken bones	Helichrysum, lavender, yarrow	Comfrey, hypericum
Fluid Retention	Angelica root, cedarwood, chamomile, juniper berry, fennel	hemp hypericum, sunflower
Heart palpitations	Angelica root, chamomile, marjoram, geranium, neroli, orange, rose, ylang-ylang	Calendula, hemp, sunflower,
Hypertension (high blood pressure)	Clary sage, lavender, neroli, ylang-ylang	Calendula, hemp, sunflower
Hypotension (low blood pressure)	Cajeput, ginger, neroli, peppermint, rosemary, thyme	Sunflower

Condition	Essential oil/ hydrosol	Carrier oil
Muscle cramps	Clary sage, juniper berry, spearmint, yarrow	Hemp, sunflower, calendula
Muscle stiffness	Cedarwood, clary sage, eucalyptus, ginger, juniper berry, lemongrass, marjoram, plai	Comfrey, hemp, hypericum
Neuro-muscular problems	Angelica root, cajeput, chamomile (Roman), peppermint, plai	Calendula, hypericum, sunflower
Edema	Angelica root, cedarwood, helichrysum, juniper berry, lemon, peppermint, rosemary, thyme	Sunflower, comfrey, calendula
Tendon Strains	Chamomile, helichrysum, lavender, peppermint, plai, spearmint, yarrow	Comfrey, calendula, neem, sunflower

Problems of the Digestive System

Condition	Essential oil/ hydrosol	Carrier oil
Anorexia/loss of appetite	Angelica Root, bergamot, carrot seed, ginger, peppermint	Hemp, sunflower
Bloating	Carrot seed, chamomile (Roman), fennel, peppermint, plai	Calendula, sunflower
Colic	Angelica Root, carrot seed, chamomile, fennel , lemongrass, neroli, orange, peppermint, plai, spearmint	Sunflower
Colitis	Carrot seed, chamomile, peppermint, plai, spearmint	Calendula, sunflower
Constipation	Fennel , ginger, orange, peppermint, seaweed	Sunflower

Condition	Essential oil/ hydrosol	Carrier oil
Diarrhea	Roman chamomile, frankincense, ginger, neroli (chronic), thyme	Calendula
Digestive Disturbances	Angelica root, chamomile, fennel, frankincense, neroli, orange, peppermint, spearmint, thyme	Calendula, hemp sunflower
Flatulence	Bergamot, fennel, ginger, spearmint	Hemp, sunflower
Food Obsessed	Bergamot, carrot seed, fennel	Sunflower
Irritable Bowel Syndrome	Carrot seed, chamomile, peppermint, plai, spearmint	Hemp, sunflower
Liver tonic	Angelica Root, carrot seed, geranium, helichrysum, juniper berry, lemon	Calendula, sunflower
Malnutrition (past and present),	Carrot seed, lemon, vetiver	Hemp, sunflower
Nausea	Chamomile, ginger, peppermint, plai, spearmint	Hemp, sunflower,
Obesity	Cedarwood, fennel, orange	Sunflower
Pancreatic Problems	Angelica root, chamomile, cedarwood, fennel, ginger	Calendula, comfrey
Sluggish Digestion	Fennel, ginger, plai, spearmint, peppermint, thyme	Hemp, sunflower
Stress Related Digestive Problems	Angelica Root, chamomile, frankincense, neroli	Hemp, sunflower
Worms	Bergamot, cajeput, carrot seed, plai, thyme	Hemp, sunflower
Ulcers	Angelica Root, frankincense, plai	Calendula, comfrey, sunflower

Condition	Essential oil/ hydrosol	Carrier oil
Underweight	Angelica root, lemon, vetiver	Hemp, sunflower

Problems of the Immune System

Allergies	Chamomile, helichrysum, yarrow	Calendula, hemp, neem
Anemia	Carrot seed, chamomile (Roman), vetiver	Hemp
Auto Immune Diseases	Angelica root, bergamot, carrot seed, chamomile, juniper berry, lemon, melissa	Hemp, hypericum, sunflower
Bacterial Infections	Bergamot, eucalyptus, ginger, helichrysum, manuka, rosalina, thyme	Calendula, comfrey, hypericum
Fever	Bergamot, cajeput, eucalyptus, rosalina	Calendula, sunflower
Immune Tonic	Angelica root, bergamot, cajeput, chamomile, eucalyptus, lemon, manuka, vetiver	Hemp, sunflower
Parvo virus	Angelica Root, cajeput, eucalyptus, ginger, lavender, lemon, manuka, rosalina, rosemary, thyme	Hemp, hypericum, sunflower
Lethargy	Cedarwood, lemon, peppermint, orange, rosemary, thyme	Hemp, sunflower
Tumors	Bergamot, fennel, frankincense	Comfrey, hemp, sunflower
Viral Infections	Bergamot, eucalyptus, helichrysum, lemon, lavender, marjoram, peppermint, rosemary	Hemp, hypericum, neem, sunflower

Condition	Essential oil/ hydrosol	Carrier oil

Problems of the Nervous System

Condition	Essential oil/ hydrosol	Carrier oil
Nerve Damage	Peppermint	Hypericum
Nerve Tonic	Angelica root, cedarwood, clary sage, lemongrass, neroli	Hypericum, sunflower
Nervous Exhaustion	Angelica root, chamomile (Roman), clary sage, helichrysum, lemon, vetiver	Hemp, hypericum, sunflower
Seizures	Clary sage, frankincense, lavender, rosemary hydrosol,	Hypericum, sunflower

Problems of the Reproductive & Endocrine System

Condition	Essential oil/ hydrosol	Carrier oil
Addison's disease	Angelica root, geranium, lemon, frankincense, peppermint	Hemp, sunflower
Cushing's Syndrome	Angelica root, geranium, peppermint	Hemp, sunflower
Irregular cycle	Sweet fennel, chamomile, geranium, rose, yarrow	Hemp, hypericum, sunflower
Genital infections	Bergamot, chamomile, lavender, manuka, rosalina	Calendula, hypericum
Hormonal Problems	Bergamot, chamomile, clary sage, geranium, fennel, rose, yarrow	hemp, hypericum, sunflower
Hypothyroidism	Geranium	Sunflower
Insufficient milk	Fennel	Comfrey, hypericum
Libido (too little)	Cedarwood, ginger, ylang-ylang	Sunflower
Libido (too much)	Ylang-ylang	Hemp, sunflower

Condition	Essential oil/ hydrosol	Carrier oil
Metabolic Syndrome	Angelica root, bergamot, carrot seed, geranium, peppermint	Hemp, hypericum, sunflower
Phantom Pregnancy	Clary Sage, fennel, geranium, peppermint, rose, vetiver, yarrow	Calendula, hypericum, sunflower
Post Parturition	Bergamot, chamomile, fennel, rose, yarrow	Calendula, sunflower
Uncomfortable heat	Clary sage, chamomile, yarrow	Calendula, hemp, hypericum

Problems of the Respiratory System

Airborne Bacteria (kills)	Bergamot, eucalyptus, thyme	
Allergies	German Chamomile, helichrysum, spearmint, yarrow	Calendula, comfrey, hemp
Asthma/wheezing	Cedarwood, clary sage, eucalyptus, frankincense, helichrysum, peppermint, plai	Comfrey, hemp, sunflower
Bronchitis	Angelica root, cajeput, eucalyptus, ginger, helichrysum, peppermint, thyme	Comfrey, hemp, sunflower
Excess Mucous	Angelica root, cedarwood, myrrh, spearmint, peppermint, thyme	Comfrey, hemp, sunflower
Infections (general respiratory)	Angelica root, cajeput, rosalina, thyme	comfrey, hemp, sunflower
Influenza	Angelica root, cajeput, eucalyptus, ginger, lavender, lemon, manuka, rosalina, rosemary, thyme	comfrey, hemp, sunflower

Condition	Essential oil/ hydrosol	Carrier oil
Kennel cough	Angelica root, bergamot, cajeput, eucalyptus, lemon, manuka, peppermint, rosalina, rosemary, thyme	comfrey, hemp, sunflower
Pneumonitis	Manuka, rosalina, thyme	Comfrey, sunflower
Recurrent Airway Obstruction (RAO, COPD)	Eucalyptus, clary sage, frankincense, helichrysum, myrrh, peppermint	Comfrey, hemp, sunflower
Sinus Problems	Cajeput, eucalyptus, ginger, lavender, peppermint, rosemary	Calendula, hemp, sunflower

Skin Problems (including nails)

Allergic Dermatitis	Bergamot, German chamomile, helichrysum	Calendula, hemp, sunflower, coconut
Alopecia (hair loss)	Carrot seed, cedarwood, chamomile, clary sage, rosemary, ylang-ylang	Hemp, sunflower
Coat (poor)	Carrot seed	Coconut, hemp,
Dandruff	Bergamot, cedarwood, geranium	Calendula, jojoba, sunflower
Eczema	Chamomile, helichrysum, lavender, yarrow	Calendula, hemp, neem, sunflower
Fungal infections	Angelica root, bergamot, cedarwood, clary sage, chamomile, fennel, geranium, helichrysum, lavender, lemon, lemongrass, manuka, myrrh, rosemary	Calendula, neem,

Condition	Essential oil/ hydrosol	Carrier oil
Flea/ Fly Repellent	Cajeput, cedarwood, eucalyptus, geranium, lavender, lemongrass, manuka, peppermint, vetiver	Neem, sunflower, grape seed
Lick granulomas	Chamomile, geranium, lavender, manuka, myrrh, rosalina, yarrow	Calendula, coconut comfrey, hypericum, neem
Hot Spots (moist dermatitis, wet eczema)	Cedarwood, chamomile, helichrysum, lavender, rosalina, thyme linalool, yarrow	Calendula, coconut sunflower
Infections	Lavender, manuka, rosalina, thyme	Calendula, comfrey, neem,
Insect Bites	Chamomile, helichrysum, lavender, yarrow	Hemp, jojoba, sunflower
Lice	Geranium, lemongrass, lavender, rosemary	Coconut, neem
Mange	Bergamot, chamomile (German), helichrysum, lavender, manuka, rosalina, thyme	Calendula, coconut, neem,
Mosquito Bites	Eucalyptus, geranium, lemongrass	Neem, calendula
Proud Flesh	Chamomile, helichrysum, lavender	Calendula, jojoba
Pyoderma	German chamomile, helichrysum, lavender, thyme linalol, yarrow	Calendula, comfrey, neem,
Ringworm	Bergamot, chamomile, helichrysum, lavender, manuka, myrrh, rosalina, thyme	Neem, calendula, coconut, jojoba,
Scars	Frankincense, lavender, neroli, yarrow	Calendula, comfrey, hypericum, jojoba

Condition	Essential oil/ hydrosol	Carrier oil
Skin Problems	Benzoin (cracked), carrot seed (poor condition) elemi (older, dry), geranium (flaky, greasy), German chamomile (eruptive), lavender, manuka (infected), myrrh (damp, oozing), Roman chamomile (stress-related, itchy), yarrow (allergic)	Calendula, coconut comfrey, hemp, hypericum, jojoba,
Soft Lumps	Angelica root, fennel, ginger, manuka	Comfrey, hemp,
Thrush	Eucalyptus, manuka, rosalina, thyme	Calendula, jojoba sunflower,
Ticks	Lemongrass, marjoram, rosalina	Neem
Tumors	Bergamot, fennel, frankincense, juniper berry, lavender, lemon	Comfrey, hemp,
Ulcers	Frankincense, manuka, rosalina, tea tree, witch hazel	Sunflower, calendula, jojoba
Rashes	German chamomile, helichrysum, lavender, yarrow	Calendula, comfrey, hemp,
Warts	Bergamot, carrot seed, lavender, tea tree	Calendula, jojoba, sunflower

Urinary System Problems

Condition	Essential oil/ hydrosol	Carrier oil
Adrenal exhaustion	Angelica root, cedarwood, frankincense, geranium, lemon, vetiver	Hypericum, sunflower
Bladder Infections	Rosalina, bergamot, cajeput, carrot seed, fennel, thyme, yarrow	Sunflower,
Bladder/kidney stones	Fennel, juniper berry, lemon	Sunflower,

Condition	Essential oil/ hydrosol	Carrier oil
Inappropriate urination	Bergamot, carrot seed, frankincense, lemon, neroli, yarrow, ylang-ylang	Hypericum sunflower,
Incontinence	Carrot seed, cedarwood, lemon, yarrow	Hemp,
Kidney Infections	Bergamot, cedarwood, chamomile, juniper berry, lemon, rosalina, thyme, yarrow	Hemp, hypericum, sunflower
Kidney Tonic	Angelica Root, bergamot, cedarwood, geranium, ginger, lemon, plai, yarrow	Hemp, sunflower

Ears & Eyes
(Caution! Do not put essential oils inside ears and eyes. Use hydrosols instead!)

Ear Infections	Chamomile, myrrh, yarrow	
Runny Eyes	Chamomile, cornflower, rose, sandalwood	
Aural Plaque	Myrrh, manuka, lavender, rosalina, thyme linalool	Calendula, neem, sunflower
Conjunctivitis	Chamomile, cornflower, rose,	
Ear Mites	Chamomile, lavender, thyme linalool	Calendula, neem
Glaucoma	Carrot seed	Sunflower, hemp

First aid

Abrasions	Helichrysum, lavender, manuka, rosalina, yarrow	Comfrey, calendula
Abscesses	Manuka, rosalina, thyme	Sunflower,

Condition	Essential oil/ hydrosol	Carrier oil
Boils	Bergamot, chamomile, helichrysum, manuka, lemon, rosalina, thyme	Calendula, jojoba
Broken Bones	Helichrysum, yarrow	Comfrey
Bruises	Helichrysum, Lavender	Comfrey, sunflower
Burns	Eucalyptus, helichrysum, lavender	Calendula, Hypericum
Cuts	Helichrysum, lavender, manuka, myrrh, rosalina, yarrow	Sunflower, jojoba, calendula,
Shock/ Hysteria	Lavender, neroli, valerian, ylang-ylang	Undiluted
Sprains & strains	Chamomile, helichrysum, marjoram, peppermint, plai, rosemary, spearmint, yarrow	Calendula, comfrey
Sunburn	Lavender, chamomile, helichrysum	Calendula, hypericum
Poisonous Bites	Angelica root, fennel, plai, thyme	Calendula, sunflower

Behavior/emotional

Abandonment	Angelica root, carrot seed, frankincense	*For behavioral*
Abuse	Angelica root, bergamot, carrot seed, helichrysum, rose, yarrow	*problems use neutral base oils, such as*
Aggression	Bergamot, hemp, clary sage, peppermint, thyme	*sunflower or grape*
Anger	Bergamot, chamomile (Roman), eucalyptus, helichrysum, rose, yarrow	*seed*

Condition	Essential oil/ hydrosol	Carrier oil
Anxiety	Chamomile, clary sage, frankincense, hemp, manuka	
Boredom	Lemon, peppermint, rosemary	
Bullying	Bergamot, peppermint, ylang-ylang	
Claustrophobic	Cajeput, clary sage, eucalyptus, frankincense	
Companion (loss)	Frankincense, neroli	
Concentration (lack of)	Cedarwood, lemon, peppermint, rosemary	
Confidence (lack of)	Cedarwood, ginger, rosemary, Ylang-ylang	
Crowds (overwhelmed by/restless in)	Angelica root, Juniper berry	
Death of companions/ dying	Frankincense, marjoram, myrrh, neroli	
Depressed	Bergamot, cypress, eucalyptus, geranium, ginger, neroli, orange, rose, thyme	
Defensive aggression	Angelica root, clary sage, frankincense, lemon, peppermint, thyme	
Disengaged	Juniper berry, myrrh, rosemary	
Erratic behavior	Bergamot, clary sage	
Fear	Angelica root, cedarwood, chamomile, frankincense, hemp, thyme, yarrow, ylang-ylang	

Condition	Essential oil/ hydrosol	Carrier oil
Flighty	Cedarwood, chamomile, neroli, vetiver	
Frustration	Bergamot, chamomile, clary sage, eucalyptus	
Hierarchical Issues	Peppermint, spearmint, ylang-ylang	
Hyperactive	Chamomile, lemon, rosemary, vetiver	
Impatient	Eucalyptus, chamomile, clary sage, helichrysum, lemon, orange	
Insecure	Angelica root, fennel, geranium, ginger, rose, vetiver	
Irritability	Bergamot, chamomile, helichrysum, peppermint, orange	
Lethargic	Bergamot, cedarwood, lemon, ginger, peppermint, rosemary, orange,	
Moodiness	Bergamot, clary sage, geranium, rose	
Nervous	Angelica root, cedarwood, chamomile, clary sage, frankincense, geranium, lavender, orange, ylang-ylang, vetiver	
New home	Cedarwood, geranium, lemon	
Obsessive behavior	Cajeput, fennel	
Pushy	Angelica root, vetiver, ylang-ylang	

Condition	Essential oil/ hydrosol	Carrier oil
Restless	Clary sage, frankincense, juniper berry, lavender, rose, valerian, vetiver, ylang-ylang	
Self Harm/ Mutilation	Angelica root, carrot seed, hemp, lemon, rose	
Separation Anxiety	Angelica root, cedarwood, frankincense, hemp, neroli, ylang-ylang	
Shy	Cedarwood, ginger, lavender, neroli, thyme, ylang-ylang	
Suspicious	Juniper berry, lemon	
Timid	Cedarwood, lavender, lemon, thyme, vetiver	
Trauma	Angelica root, rose, yarrow	
Travel Phobia	Frankincense, ginger, neroli, peppermint, spearmint	
Worry	Fennel, lavender, lemon, frankincense, myrrh, peppermint, spearmint	

GLOSSARY OF TERMS

Amenorrhoea	Absence of menstruation
Anaemia	Deficiency in either quality or quantity of red blood corpuscles
Anesthetic	Substance causing loss of feeling or sensation
Analgesic	Relieves pain without producing anesthesia
Anaphrodisiac	Reduces sexual desire
Anodyne	Stills pain and quiets disturbed feelings
Antacid	Counteracts or neutralizes acidity (usually in the stomach)
Anthelmintic	Destroys intestinal worms
Antiallergenic	Relieves or controls allergic symptoms
Antianemic	Prevents or cures anaemia
Anti anxiety	Prevents or cures anxiety
Antiarthritic	Prevents or cures arthritis
Antibacterial	Destroys bacteria or inhibits their growth
Anticatarrhal	Relieves inflammation of the mucous membranes in the head, and reduces the production of mucous.
Anticoagulant	Prevents or stops the blood clotting
Anticonvulsant	Stops, prevents or lessons convulsions/seizures
Antidepressant	Prevents or cures depression
Antiemetic	Reduces nausea/vomiting
Antifungal	Destroys or prevents the growth of fungi
Antihistamine	Used to treat allergies because it counteracts the effects of histamine such as swelling, congestion, sneezing and itchy eyes.

Anti-inflammatory	Reduces inflammation
Antilactogenic	Reduces milk production
Antineuralgic	Relieves neuralgia (nerve pain), an acute, intermittent pain that radiates along a nerve.
Antioxidant	Antioxidants are substances that prevent or slow oxidation to prevent cell damage.
Antiparasitic	Kills or inactivates parasites
Antiphlogistic	Reduces inflammation
Antipruritic	Relieves itching
Antirheumatic	Relieves rheumatism
Antisclerotic	Prevents hardening of tissue
Anti seborrhea	Prevents the abnormal secretion and discharge of sebum, which gives the skin an oily appearance and forms greasy scales.
Antiseptic	Inhibits the growth and reproduction of microorganisms, when applied to the body they reduce the possibility of infection, sepsis or putrefaction.
Antispasmodic	Prevents/eases spasms or convulsions
Antisudorific	Prevents or inhibits sweating/perspiration
Antitoxic	Counteracts a toxin or poison
Antitussive	Inhibits the cough reflex helping to stop coughing
Antiviral	Inhibits growth of a virus
Aperient	Mildly laxative
Aphrodisiac	Increases sexual desire
Arthritis	Inflammation of joints
Astringent	Causes contraction of organic tissues, control of bleeding, styptic
Bactericidal	Kills bacteria
Calmative	Mildly sedative, relaxing
Cardio-tonic	Strengthens and invigorates the heart
Carminative	Reduces flatulence, settles digestive system
Cephalic	Diseases affecting the head/remedy for disorders of the brain

Cholagogue	Stimulates secretion of flow of bile into duodenum
Choleretic	Stimulates the production of bile by the liver
Cicatrizant	Promotes formation of scar tissue, aids healing
Concrete	Waxy concentrated solid or semi-solid perfume material, prepared from live plant matter
Decongestant	Relieves congestion, usually by reducing the swelling of the mucous membranes in the nasal passages.
Deodorant	Masks or suppresses odors
Detoxicant	Removes toxins – substances which have a harmful chemical nature
Digestive Stimulant	Stimulates digestion
Digestive Tonic	Strengthens and invigorates digestion
Diuretic	Aids production of flow of urine
Emmenagogue	Induces menstruation
Emollient	Softens, soothes and lubricates the skin
Energizing	Invigorates and gives energy
Enuresis	Urinary incontinence
Euphoric	Exaggerated feeling of well being or elation
Expectorant	Promotes clearing of chest/lungs
Febrifuge	Combats fever, antipyretic
Fortifying	Strengthening
Glandular Tonic	Strengthens and invigorates the glands
Hemostatic	Stops bleeding
Hepatic	Any compound that acts on the liver
Hormone-like	Acts like a hormone
Hydrosol/hydrolat	bi-product from essential oil distillation
Hyperglycemic	Having excessively high blood sugar
Hypoglycemic	Having excessively low blood sugar
Hypertensive	Raises blood pressure
Hypo-uricemic	Breaks down uric acid
Hypotensive	Lowers blood pressure
Immune Tonic	Strengthens and invigorates the immune system

Immunostimulant	Stimulates various functions or activities of the immune system
Infusion	Herbs etc steeped in liquid to extract soluble constituents
Insect Repellent	Repels insects
Insecticide	Kills insects
Kidney Tonic	Strengthens and invigorates the kidneys
Lactogenic	Enhances milk production
Laxative	Moves the bowels and aids digestion
Leucocyte-stimulant	Increases the production of leukocytes, white blood cells, part of the immune system
Limbic system	A group of interconnected deep brain structures, common to all mammals, and involved in olfaction, emotion, motivation, behavior, and various autonomic functions.
Litholytic	An agent that dissolves urinary calculi (stones)
Macerated oil	Infusion of herbs in vegetable oil
Mucolytic	Dissolves mucous
Nervine:	Having a soothing effect on the nerves
Neurotonic	Strengthens and invigorates the nerves
Estrogen-Like	Has a similar effect on the body to that of estrogen
Olfactory system	The parts of the body involved in sensing smell, including the nose and many parts of the brain
Pancreatic-stimulant	Increases pancreatic activity
Parasiticide	Destroys parasites internally and externally
Pathogenic	Causing or producing disease
Pathological	Unnatural or destructive process on living tissue
Phlebotonic	Having a toning action on the veins
Purgative	Strongly laxative
Pyorrhea	Bleeding or discharge of pus
Regenerative	Restores or revives tissue growth
Reproductive stimulant	Increases reproductive activity in the body
Restorative	Restores health or strength

Rubefacient	Causes redness of skin, possibly irritation
Sedative	Reduces excitability and calms
Sexual Tonic	Strengthens and invigorates the sexual function
Smooth Muscle Relaxant	Relaxes the smooth muscles, which are muscles that contract without conscious control and are found in the walls of internal organs such as stomach, intestine and bladder.
Soothing	Brings comfort or relief
Soporific	Sleep inducing
Stimulant	Increases physiological or nervous activity in the body/ promotes activity, interest or enthusiasm.
Stomachic	Promotes digestion or appetite
Styptic	Astringent, stops bleeding
Sudorific	Diaphoretic, produces sweat
Tincture	Alcoholic solution of some (usually vegetable) principle used in medicine
Tonic	Produces or restores normal vigor or tension (tone)
Uterine Tonic	Strengthens and invigorates the uterus
Vasodilator	Widens or dilates blood vessels
Vermifuge	Expels intestinal worms, anthelmintic
Vesicant	Causes blistering to skin, a counter-irritant by external application
Vulnerary	Promotes healing of wounds

Resources

Videos of dogs interacting with essential oils
Subtle response video,
https://www.youtube.com/watch?v=7qtKzNk4m2o
Expressive response,
https://www.youtube.com/watch?v=nb9GCRYXG-k
Dog selecting essential oils,
https://www.youtube.com/watch?v=hhq773D0KNI
For dog training and behavior advice
http://www.patriciamcconnell.com/behavior-and-health

Books
So many books, so little time, but here are a few I have enjoyed.

Aromatics
Aromatherapy for Healing the Spirit, *Gabriel Mojay*
Aromatherapy for Health professionals, *Shirley Price and Len Price*
Carrier Oils, *Len Price, with Ian Smith and Shirley Price*
Essential Oil Safety: Second Edition, *Robert Tisserand*
Hydrosols, The Next Aromatherapy, *Suzanne Catty*
Medical Aromatherapy: Healing with Essential Oils, *Kurt Schnaubelt*

The Chemistry of Aromatherapeutic Oils, *E.Joy Bowles*
The Complete Guide to Aromatherapy, *Salvatore Battaglia*
The Encyclopedia of Essential Oils, *Julia Lawless*
Understanding Hydrolats: The specific hydrosols for aromatherapy, *Len and Shirley Price*

Dog health and behavior

Give Your Dog a Bone: The Practical Common Sense Way to Feed Dogs For a Long Healthy Life, *Ian Billinghurst*

What's for dinner Dexter, Cooking for your pets, *Judy Morgan*

Healthy Dogs, Your Loving Touch, *Sherri Cappabianca*

Natural Nutrition For Dogs & Cats: The Ultimate Diet, *Kymythy Schultze*

Wild Health, How animals keep themselves well and what we can learn from them, *Cindy Engel*

Four Paws Five Directions, *Cheryl Schwartz, DVM*

The truth About Dogs, *Stephen Budiansky*

Understanding and handling dog aggression, *Barbara Sykes*

How to speak dog, *Stanley Coren*

The APBC book of companion animal behavior, *edited by David Appleby*

Animal minds, by Donald R. Griffin

Dogs misbehaving, *by Martin J. Scott and Gael Mariani*

Anything written by Patricia McConnell

Suppliers

There are many quality suppliers of aromatics, these are some I have sampled and like. It is not a comprehensive list. Just because someone is not on it does not mean their oils are not good, simply that I have not tried them.

USA

Eden Botanicals
Floracopeia
Aromatics International
Nature's Gift
Stillpoint Aromatics
White Lotus Aromatics

Europe

Kobashi
Materia Aromatica
Florihana
Oshadhi
Norfolk Essential oils
Wild Health Shop

About Nayana

Nayana Morag grew up in the UK in a large family of humans and animals, the perfect environment for learning about animal behavior. She was one of those kids with a natural empathy for animals, always gravitating towards the needy and vulnerable.

By the age of 18 she had developed an interest in natural health and complementary medicines and had started to travel widely, learning about everything from horse care to Hippocrates as she went.

Nayana was introduced to Caroline Ingraham the pioneer of using essential oils with zoopharmacognosy in 1997. From the first time she saw a horse select an essential oil she was hooked. Nayana earned her Certificate in Animal Aromatherapy and Touch for Health for Animals in 1999 and has been practicing her art ever since.

Over the years, Nayana has developed a system of animal wellness that incorporates aromatics, Traditional Chinese Medicine, and reducing stress through management and diet. She calls her system Animal PsychAromatica and offers courses at all levels to students around the world. If you have any queries or comments about the book or would like to learn from Nayana, you can reach her through www.essentialanimals.com

CPSIA information can be obtained
at www.ICGtesting.com
Printed in the USA
BVHW01s1054121217

502434BV00004B/148/P